Guiding Yoga's Light

Guiding Yoga's Light

Yoga Lessons for Yoga Teachers

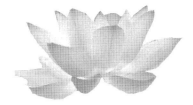

Nancy Gerstein, RYT

Pendragon Publishing, Inc.
Chicago

Guiding Yoga's Light

ISBN 0-9722809-8-7 (trade paper)

Library of Congress Cataloging-in-Publication Data:

Gerstein, Nancy, 1958-
 Guiding yoga's light : yoga lessons for yoga teachers / Nancy Gerstein.
    p. cm.
 Includes bibliographical references and index.
  ISBN 0-9722809-8-7 (pbk.)
 1. Hatha yoga—Study and teaching. I. Title.

RA781.7.G44 2004
 613.7'046'071—dc22

                    2004016578

Edited and Layout by Kate Palandech (K²P)

Printed in the United States of America
Pendragon Publishing, Inc.
P.O. Box 31665
Chicago, IL 60631
www.pendragonpublishinginc.com

For Dave, Max and Grace,
the lights of my life.

Be a lamp to yourself.

Be your own confidence.

Hold on to the truth within yourself as to the only truth.

Buddha

Contents

Acknowledgments

This work would not be possible without the guidance of the many yogis who came before me. I humbly thank Swami Rama and all the teachings he has most graciously imparted through his books and lectures, as well as the remarkably spirited and generous teachers he has trained.

I'd also like to thank Sandra Anderson and Rolf Solvik who are the "real deal," the truest of yogis I have ever met. Thank you for your scholarly brilliance, your compassion, and the insight into the Himalayan teachings you have so effortlessly interpreted and passed along.

Thank you to Kate Palandech at Pendragon Publishing, who took a chance on this yogi. I thank you for all your *chakras*, but especially the third one.

Thank you to my first teachers, my mother Bobbie and father Louie; my sister Judy and brother-in-law Allan for their unconditional love and support; to my brother Donny for his legal eyes; and to Judith for her sagely editorial advice.

Special thanks to all at the Himalayan Institute Midwest for the use of their beautiful space in which to photograph our *asanas*.

From the bottom of this yogi's heart, I most gratefully thank all of my teaching companions, yoga students (many of whom have been *my* greatest teachers) and lifelong friends, Marcie and Mindy for helping me realize my life's passion and purpose.

For Dave, my outer light and spiritual mentor. Sometimes the best advice is staring us in the face. Thanks for being the face of wisdom.

Finally, to Max and Grace who have the cutest little *asasas* I know.

Let us rise up and be thankful,

for if we didn't learn a lot today, at least we learned a little,

and if we didn't learn a little, at least we didn't get sick,

and if we got sick, at least we didn't die;

so, let us all be thankful.

Buddha

"I must have wandered upon this path for a reason. Maybe it was a quick reminder to catch my breath or stretch my hamstrings or look upon a furious driver with compassion. I now know there are thousands of lessons to be learned from the school of yoga."

Anonymous Yoga Student

Introduction

What is this love affair we have with yoga? The practice itself is time-consuming and laborious, but it is also serendipitous and exciting. A wonderfully curious adventure, it is a momentous discovery, a quiet day trip into our inner world with each instant on our yogic path holding the opportunity to feel spacious, connected and alive.

Since the beginning of my yoga journey, I have cherished how the ancient teachings apply to every aspect of modern living; from our jobs, to our relationships, to raising our kids, to running errands, to grieving our loved ones, the lessons of yoga are found everywhere. Perhaps this love affair with yoga is grounded in the eternal love of life itself.

Guiding Yoga's Light is a starting point, a tool for bringing the wealth of the yoga experience into the daily lives of both teachers and students. Over a period of years I have recorded my various lesson plans as a means of keeping track of where I've been as a teacher and where the yogic path has taken me as a student. These lesson plans have proved to be a rewarding guide motivating me in one direction or another, and helping me focus my intentions on my own practice.

It is not my objective to make all yoga programs alike, but rather to offer a template to help explore each yoga lesson wherever it may lead. Armed with the knowledge that our yoga ancestors have provided us, I feel we must continually seek to create a yoga experience that is both vital and current to our modern day students while keeping the traditional meanings intact. It is with great joy and love in my heart that I venture this text as a very tiny step toward meeting that end.

Your yoga begins when you leave the classroom.

It's how you relate to people and how you relate to the world.

Your yoga is the giving and receiving.

It's the wellness between inner and outer worlds.

Your yoga is living the purpose of your life.

Your yoga is to spread peace, one person at a time.

The light and love in me

bows to light and love in you.

Om

Shanti. Shanti. Shanti.

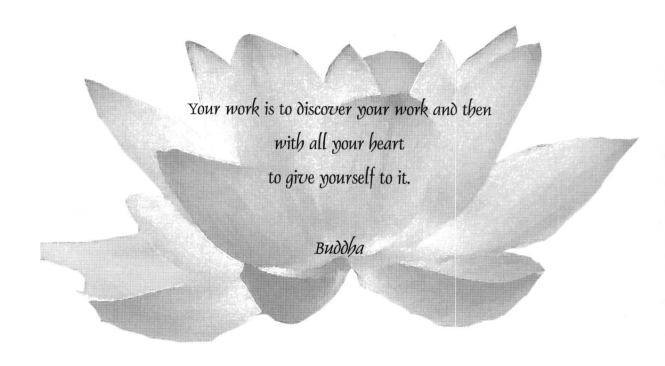

Your work is to discover your work and then
with all your heart
to give yourself to it.

Buddha

Eight Limbs of *Raja* Yoga

Raja means "royal" and deliniates the path of Yoga in the highest, most comprehensive form.

Gathered by the sage, Patanjali Maharishi, in his *Yoga Sutras*, the Eight Limbs are a progressive series of steps or disciplines which purify the body, mind and spirit, leading the yogi to enlightenment and liberation from suffering.

Limb One — *Yamas* The Restraints

Ahimsa — non-violence

Satya — truthfulness

Asteya — non-stealing

Brahmacharya — moderation in all things

Aparigraha — non-possessiveness

Limb Two — *Niyamas* Observances

Saucha — purity

Santosha — contentment

Tapas — austerity and self-discipline

Svadhyaya — self-study

Ishvara Pranidhana — surrender to divine consciousness

The Eight Limbs of *Raja* Yoga (continued)

Limb Three — *Asana*

posture

Limb Four — *Pranayama*

regulation or control of prana

Limb Five — *Pratyahara*

withdrawal of the senses

Limb Six — *Dharana*

concentration

Limb Seven — *Dhyana*

meditation

Limb Eight — *Samadhi*

super-conscious state

How to Use the Lessons

Each lesson in *Guiding Yoga's Light* consists of six key elements:

1) Intention. Sets up the meaning of the day's class. Allows students to derive meaning from their yoga experience.

2) Approximate Time. The length of each written lesson. If you want to add or edit the lesson please note that any changes or added pauses will change the approximate length of the script.

3) The Lesson. The core of your class; it is the essence of the day's teaching. From this core come the next three information blocks to help enhance your class.

4) *Asanas* for Deepening. Suggested *asanas* that illustrate through body stretch, movement, and sensation how to feel the lesson within the body. These are *suggested asanas*, please be sure to include the *asanas* that work best for your teaching practice.

5) Practice off the Mat. May be used as a "homework" assignment, reminder, or topic for discussion to keep the lessons of yoga on top of your students' minds.

6) Wise Words. Include quotes, quips and other suggestions to engage your students within the context of the lesson.

Tips from the Front of the Room

1) Do your best to have a relaxed presence. Until you feel calm and centered, think of yourself as both student and teacher.

2) Enjoy the day's lesson. Discover what it means to you so you can put your heart into it.

3) Teach what you need to learn. There's more passion and benefit for those you teach.

4) Don't compare yourself to others, including other teachers. Everyone has their own light that they shine uniquely.

5) Teaching is a joy and a privilege. It is your path and your profession to help others find healing, space, and inner peace. Make every moment count.

Publisher's note: *Guiding Yoga's Light* was specifically designed to be a *worked* book — crack the spine so it lays flat, write in the *Notes* columns and around the *Asanas* photographs, bend the side flaps to hold your favorite spot. Enjoy making it your yoga practice's workbook!

Chapter One

Words have the power to both destroy and heal.

When words are both true and kind, they can change our world.

Buddha

Beginning Lessons

During the first few weeks with your new class, you, as the yogic guide, have much to teach your students.

• **For new yogis** the primary focus is on *asana* — postures — and opening the outermost layer of the body. This opening, strengthening and ultimately aligning of the body, clears the subtle energy channels or *nadis*. This cleansing enhances the flow of *prana* — lifeforce.

Guided by mind and breath, the enhanced flow of *prana* creates changes on all levels —physical, emotional and spiritual. Most students feel the effects of their practice the very first time on the mat.

• **For experienced yogis** practice profoundly effects mental and spiritual layers by both calming the mind and awakening substantial intelligence throughout the body. As yogis, we experience a deeper knowing into our essential nature and the world. The practice becomes a quintessential ingredient on the path to living a more fulfilling, healthier, and awakened life.

Whether your class consists of new *or* experienced yogis, please consider the following points when structuring your lesson plans:

• *Hatha* **Yoga is not just an exercise system**. It's a 5,000-year old holistic path of health and self-development that begins with the body as a tangible way to affect all aspects of our being.

• **Never underestimate breath awareness**. The breath is the link between body and mind. Demonstrate and teach the practice during every class. Mindful breathing during class can mean the difference between achieving the holistic effects of *asana* and simply stretching.

• **Practice is both individualistic and systematic**. Encourage students to challenge themselves in an effort to begin the process of change, but not to go into a zone of pain. There should never be any striving or forcing of *asana* or breath. Integral in the practice is acceptance of body as we find it, in the present, moment to moment.

• **Beginner's mind/open mind**. Remind students that every day on the yoga mat is new and different. As Japanese Zen monk, Suzuki said, "In the beginner's mind there are many possibilities, in the expert's mind there are few."

• **Have fun with your lesson plans**. Teach the lessons *you* want to learn. This insures your lessons come from the heart.

First Class Facts

Intention: To give beginning students the foundation of yoga.
Approximate Length: 3-4 minutes

Hello, and welcome to the ancient science of yoga. Before we begin, I want to go over a few things you should know to make your experience in yoga class the best it can be.

• Yoga is practiced in bare feet, so please take off your shoes and socks. Our feet have tiny little receptors on the bottom so when our feet are bare, we can feel the earth beneath us and it helps improve our balance.
• Come to class with an empty stomach. Wait about 2 to 3 hours after a big meal, about an hour after a snack.
• Please turn off your cellphones and pagers.
• Try to come to class a few minutes early. Consider being prompt as part of your practice.
• Let me know of any pre-existing injury or special conditions so I can help you.
• Do your best to let go of any competitive mind-set with yourself or with others. Yoga is absolutely non-competitive. It's not just a work-out; it's a spiritual practice that makes the body stronger, more flexible, and generally much healthier. But the aim is to calm the mind, open the heart, and stimulate your own spiritual evolution.

Within the last few years, the practice of yoga has been praised for its stress reducing capabilities. Basically, it works like this: stress and tension cause the body to tighten up. Tension literally blocks off the energy flow.

In yoga, we use the *asanas*—postures, and the breath to learn to open

Notes

every constricted area of the body and mind. This helps to release and erase tension. As the body relaxes and opens, the mind also becomes calm and less busy.

When the mind is less busy, negative feelings such as anxiety, fear and anger melt away. The mind then begins to open up to things like patience, acceptance and compassion.

Practicing yoga is a healing process. It's not about getting poses picture-perfect, it's about being sensitive to your own body and quiet enough to hear your own inner voice.

The one ground rule we have is to please stay within your physical limitations. This means listening carefully to what your body is telling you and honoring its messages, erring on the side of safety. If you want to grow and heal, you have to take responsibility for listening to yourself.

And most of all, have fun. This should feel good!

It is recommended this script be followed with an introduction into diaphragmatic breathing.

Asanas for Deepening

Reclining twists
Leg cradles
Reclining hamstring stretch
Shoulder stretches

Practice off the Mat

Keep your mind on what you're doing. When your mind wanders off to work, worries, or responsibilities, bring it back to the moment.

Notes

Wise Words

Listen to your inner teacher. He/she has much to teach you.

The body's language is sensation. Listen to what the body tells you.

Yoga is a time-tested path for developing a deeper experience of yourself and the world.

Be kind and loving to yourself by accepting yourself just as you are.

Many of us are physically stressed because we believe our minds and bodies are separate.

Asanas

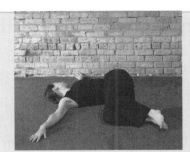

Reclining Twist-
knee over knee

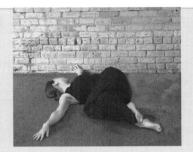

Reclining Twist-
eagle legs

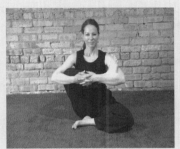

Leg Cradle

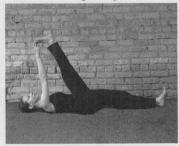

Reclining Hamstring
Stretch

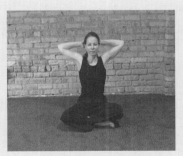

Shoulder Stretch

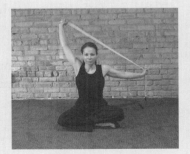

Shoulder Stretch

Notes

Learning Diaphragmatic Breathing

Intention: To illustrate and educate students on the value of diaphragmatic breathing.
Approximate Time: 6-8 minutes

The very foundation of our yoga practice is to learn to breathe properly and completely. We refer to this as breathing from our diaphragm or diaphragmatic breathing. Diaphragmatic breathing allows us to slow down our heart rate, bring our blood pressure down, clear our minds and relax our muscles. In fact, it's the single most important thing we can do to offset everyday stress.

When we're *not* breathing fully, our blood pressure goes up, heart rate is increased, our muscles get tense, and even our thinking becomes scattered.

Breathing properly is not just the foundation of yoga, it's the foundation of life itself. It's the very first thing we do when we're born, it's the last thing we do when we die. You can live a few weeks without food, but only a few minutes without breathing!

So let's learn diaphragmatic breathing.

Begin in *shavasana*, feet about 12 inches apart, arms at your sides, palms up.

Take a moment and leave any thoughts outside that do not belong right here in this room. Sweep those thoughts outside of this room. Leave your past and your future, stay right here in the present; don't let go. This is your time to look inward and take care of your well-being. In doing so, you'll be better equipped to handle the challenges that life throws your way.

Close your eyes and focus on your breath. Bring all your awareness to your breathing, breathing through the nose. Notice if your breathing is shallow or noisy. Is your inhale the same length as your exhale?

Bring your focus to the space between your nostrils. Feel the coolness of the inhale, the warmth of the exhale. By focusing here, you're starting to turn inside.

The idea here is to slide into awareness of the breath. Gently. No forcing. No pushing. Just remain present to the coming and going of breath. When the mind wanders off to work, family or responsibilities, simply bring it back to the breath. Back to the breath.

Now we're going to make sure we're breathing completely from our diaphragm. First, soften the belly — consciously release any tension you may be holding there. Then, put your right hand on your abdomen and put your left hand on your chest. To breathe diaphragmatically, your right hand should be moving up and down so that your abdomen naturally extends out a bit on the inhale and goes back down on the exhale. Your left hand should be relatively still. (Pause long enough for students to take 3 to 5 breaths.) If only your left hand is moving, you're chest-breathing and getting about one-third to one-half of the oxygen you'd be getting from breathing through your diaphragm.

If you're not getting it today, just keep trying. We're going to breathe diaphragmatically from our nose throughout class. By breathing through a posture, it helps us relax through it.

The deeper you breathe, the more relaxed and focused you become. Never forget to breathe.

Every inhale brings in fresh *prana* or lifeforce. Every exhale releases toxins and tensions of the day.

Being sensitive to the whole body, we breathe in, being sensitive to the whole body, we breathe out.

No striving, no forcing.

Notes

Notes

Asanas for Deepening

Sitting Side Stretch to open the intercostal muscles between the ribs.
Sitting Clam (forward bend in an easy pose)
Makarasana **(crocodile)**. Feel breath fill the lower back.
Uttanasana **(standing forward bend)**. Sense how the breath vibrates the torso.

Practice off the Mat

Practice diaphragmatic breathing for 5 minutes a day, either in *shavasana* or crocodile. Once you're able to use the diaphragmatic breath to keep emotions in balance, you'll immediately discover the value of breath awareness.

Wise Words

Gently nudge your tight areas with breath.

Diaphragmatic breathing is innate. Babies do it without any training. Later in life, when stress sneaks into our consciousness, we forget how.

Yoga is preparation for living. It gives us a curiosity and enthusiasm to participate in life.

The breath is the link between body and mind.

Asanas

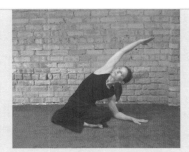

Sitting Side Stretch

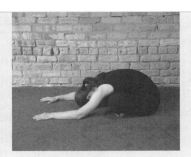

Clam

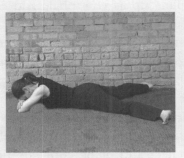

Makarasana
crocodile

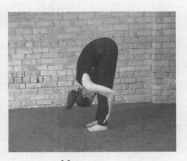

Uttanasana
standing forward bend

Notes

Benefits of Yoga

Intention: To create awareness of the benefits of yoga practice.
Approximate Time: 2 minutes

Lie in *shavasana*, feet about 12 inches apart, arms at your sides, palms up. Rock your head side-to-side until you find the flat part on your skull, and rest your head there.

Feel your abdomen rise and fall with each breath. Imagine your lungs as a pair of balloons — filling up as you inhale and emptying out as you exhale. As they fill, they become longer and rounder — they grow in all directions. You begin to feel the air going into your back, into the chest, sideways down the waist, every breath elongating the spine.

• Yoga is a practical philosophy involving every aspect of our being. It teaches us both self-discipline and self-awareness.

• At the physical level, it gives us relief from illness. The postures strengthen and stretch the body and create a feeling of well-being.

• Yoga sharpens the intellect and helps concentration.

• Our breathing practices calm the mind.

• Spiritually, yoga introduces us to inner awareness and gives us the gift of being still.

The whole path of yoga is a journey of attaining inner peace. Let's begin the journey.

Asanas for Deepening

Rocking Chair. Enhances spinal awareness.

Cat Stretch. Put awareness in the whole body — from the top of the head to the soles of the feet. Take the time to move with the breath, inhaling the breath at the navel center and sending it through the body on exhale.

Reclining Hip Openers

Practice off the Mat

Notice the subtle changes happening in your life. Do you sleep better after your yoga practice? Are you more aware of your breath and how it may relate to your emotions?

Wise Words

See what every posture has to teach you.

Listen to the sound of your breath, feel it in every cell, imagine that the breath is stretching you.

Next time you're in a tense situation, consciously relax your shoulders and establish your diaphragmatic breath. Notice the positive effects of actively working stress out of your body.

Every emotion puts its imprint on our physcial body.

Notes

Asanas

Rocking Chair

Cat Stretch

Reclining Hip Openers

reclining easy pose   reclining leg cradle

Softening the Edges

Notes

Intention: To train the body and mind to surrender to the practice.
Approximate Time: 2-3 minutes

Lie in *shavasana.* Take a few minutes to relax and settle the body, especially the abdominal area. Then gently bring your attention to rest on your breath.

Allow the breath to be loose and unrestricted. With each exhalation, feel the weight of the body surrender to the floor, allowing every muscle to release its grip on the bones. Feel the eyes relax and soften and all the facial muscles release.

During today's practice, keep the definition of yoga or union on top of your mind. This is about being integrated and connecting our breath, body and mind. From this integration comes liberation, and *that's* when yoga happens.

The breath leads this connection. So by staying linked with the breath, we may direct *prana* or lifeforce into areas that are tight, shallow or shut down.

We can then slowly and mindfully build an *asana* out of the breath's vibration, letting the breath move us.

When you work with this purpose, the pose becomes alive, easy and fluid, not forced or stiff or out-of-breath. Tight edges gently soften.

Roughness or shortness of breath is a symptom that you're forcing instead of softening first and letting the breath do it's job. So instead of getting yourself into an *asana*, first get into the breath and then flow with it into the *asana*. Let your breath be your partner. Become one with it.

Let's try it. Follow your in-breath and out-breath. Connect with the breath before you begin to move your body.

Notes

Asanas for Deepening

Reclining Side Stretch. Soften the ribs and each side of the back to help relax into the postures that follow.

Twisting Triangle. Stretch legs apart 3-4 feet. Line up the toes and heels. Bring one hand to the floor, opposite arm reaches toward the sky. Soften the pose one breath at a time. Welcome the subtle openings from hamstrings to shoulders, from heels to fingertips.

Standing *Yoga Mudra*. Enjoy pouring your body toward the floor. Drain the tension out of the shoulders and upper back.

Practice off the Mat

Every time you say something to yourself that's negative, it has a tiny but measurable negative effect on your body. Think about what you think as well as what you say.

Wise Words

Keep your posture inventive — recreate it over and over if necessary.

Give your muscles permission to soften and lengthen.

Accept where you are in this moment. Acceptance is the ingredient that can make change possible.

Get your lines long. Then lengthen those lines without collapsing or making the pose stiff or dull.

Acknowledge rather than resist your limitations. Tell yourself, "It's OK to be just who I am."

Asanas

Reclining Side Stretch

Twisting Triangle

Standing *Yoga Mudra*

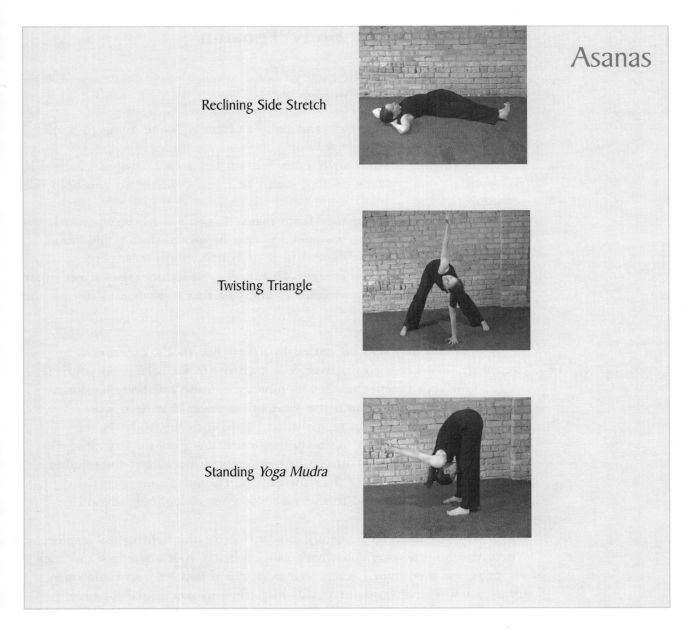

Body Tension

Notes

Intention: Discovering the roots of our tension.
Approximate Length: 3-4 minutes

Today, through breath and body awareness, we're going to work with and through our body tension.

In the yogic perspective, every tension has a cause that lies behind it. Ask yourself today what's causing *you* to be tense? Where do you hold this tension?

Tension could originate from many things: a relationship, work, anger, fatigue, caffeine, even something that happened during childhood. Muscle tension blocks the natural flow of lymph, hormones, nerve impulses, blood and *pranic* energy. Eventually, these blockages affect other parts of the body creating weaknesses and lowering resistance to disease and infection.

It's the ripple effect.

Tension may also be caused by excess like foods, exercise, work, even rest. The key is to discover your own needs for balance in your life.

Our yoga practice teaches us how we can use our body tension as a learning tool to guide us into the areas of ourselves that need work.

Let's now lie down in *shavasana*. Tune into the body on the ground. Feel the parts of the body that touch the ground. Pay close attention to the breath. This can be very difficult because if the mind is busy, it moves much faster than the breath. The breath may feel awkwardly slow compared to the speed of your thoughts. Acknowledge this without judging.

In your mind's eye, gently look inside for the tight areas: explore where you hold tension and what's causing it. If your shoulders and neck are tight, ask them why. Keep your eyes closed and let your mind open up — a few simple words or visuals may come to you. Take the time to look clearly to see what's there.

Asanas For Deepening

Practice approaching poses with tension. For instance, go into trikonasana (triangle) with exaggerated shoulder tension. Then, slowly take the tension out.

Naukasana (reclining boat). Releases a central acupressure point located between the navel and the breastbone. Long deep breathing in this pose helps free body tension.
Shoulder Openers. Eagle arms, arm swings, and tense and release exercises.
Neck stretches. Side-to-side, looking over one shoulder then the other, chin to chest.
Gomukhasana (cow's face). Allow the hips to settle. Frustration and anger are often lodged in the hip area. Notice what happens when you tune into tension and consciously release it.

Practice off the Mat

Be open and receptive for all the other benefits of yoga to come at anytime during your day.

Watch your anger factor. Uncontrolled emotions can use up a great deal of energy. A few minutes of anger can use more energy than a day of physical labor.

Wise Words

The pose should feel bright and light, otherwise it becomes heavy and clogged.

Change will happen once the mind's ability to control has been removed.

Notes

Asanas

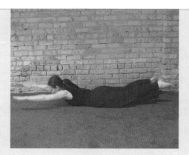

Naukasana
boat

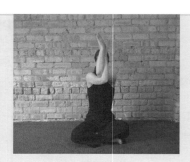

Eagle Arms

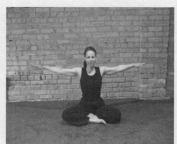

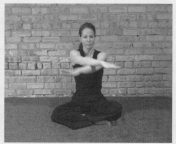

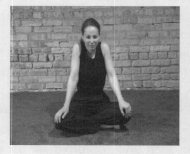

arm swing wide

Shoulder Openers
arm swing cross

tense and release

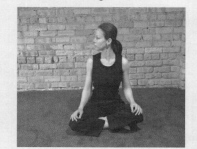

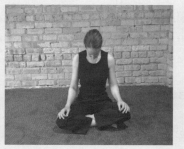

Neck Stretches

Gomukhasana
cow's face

Lengthening the Exhalation

Notes

Intention: To learn the art of relaxation during stressful life situations.
Approximate Time: 3 minutes

Beginning Movements: Neck and shoulder stretches.

Lie in *shavasana*. Take a few minutes to relax and settle the body. Then gently bring your attention to rest on your exhalation, following the exhalation all the way down into the pause at the end at the breath. Calmly focus on watching your breath for a few minutes.

With each exhalation, feel the weight of the body surrendering to the floor, allowing every muscle to release its grip on the bones. Then, very, very gradually begin to lengthen your exhalation. If you feel any shortness of breath, back off a bit. The extension of breath should feel natural. Open your mouth if this helps.

Continue on until you find a comfortable rhythm where you feel relaxed and calm. As you enter a deeper state of relaxation, let go of any control of your breathing and simply watch the spontaneous breathing pattern that's happening.

Notice how you feel right now. Does the mind feel clearer? Do the muscles feel relaxed? Note that this ability to consciously relax yourself is only a few exhalations away.

Let's use this gift of lengthening the exhale to facilitate healing in today's practice.

Asanas for Deepening
Notice the cleansing power of the exhalation with each asana.

Adho Mukha Shvanasana (**downdog**). Move into the posture with long exhale.

Janu Shirshasana (head-to-knee). Exhale and fold forward — do this several times. As you inhale, feel the chest opening and lifting away from the pelvis. Feel any tight or stuck spots and breathe into those places, releasing tension with the out-breath.

Practice off the Mat

During stressful times, feel the tension leaving your body, releasing all its toxins, darkness and unwanted emotions with each consciously long exhalation.

Wise Words

Not knowing how long we stay in the pose forces us stay in the moment — a practice that leads to a sense of peace and happiness.

By being consciously attentive to the thoughts and sensations, we understand that the mind constantly influences *asana*.

Scan your body and find out where you feel stuck, open, strong or weak.

Asanas

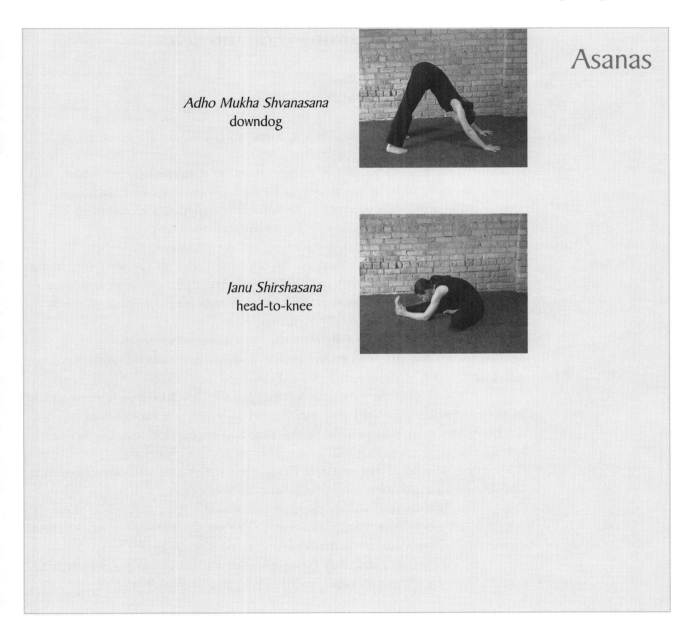

Adho Mukha Shvanasana
downdog

Janu Shirshasana
head-to-knee

Defining *Ha* and *Tha*

Intention: To define *Hatha* Yoga.
Approximate Time: 2-3 minutes

The balance of body, breath, mind and spirit is not an easy one. From day to day, minute to minute, we may find ourselves emotionally swinging back and forth. But it's with a calm and relaxed state of body and mind that we're able to *accept* and *adapt* to life's changes and challenges. This is an essential component to living a more joyous and balanced life.

Hatha Yoga is fundamentally all about balance.

The definition of yoga is union, yoking or joining together. *Ha* means sun and *tha* means moon — or opposites, and all the attributes that go with these opposites: hot and cold, dark and light, physical and mental, male and female. *Hatha* yoga is the union of opposites in order to reach balance — mentally, physically, spiritually.

Hatha Yoga is referred to as the physical practice of doing the postures with the proper breathing that *leads* to harmony of body, breath, mind and spirit.

It's said that the postures were originally developed as a prerequisite to concentration *(dharana)* and meditation *(dhyana)*. To the ancient yogis, the body was seen as a vehicle to the soul and meditation was the key to getting there. However, to sit in meditation for long periods of time, the body must be free of tension and flexible enough to sit without discomfort. The mind must be quiet and able to concentrate.

The body is the vehicle to the soul, so treat it with respect. Feel your boundaries. Sense your limitations. But on all levels of consciousness, expect and allow yourself to expand.

(Seated or in *shavasana*) Bring all your awareness to your breathing, establishing the diaphragmatic breath. Feel your abdomen rise

Notes

and fall with each breath. Observe the natural flow of breath in and out of your body. Let the breath be the link between the mind and the body.

Asanas For Deepening

Remember to balance the ha and tha by practicing easy with challenging, relaxing with invigorating, stretching with strengthening.

Serpent. Press the toes toward the forehead. Note the difference in stretching one side and the other.
Vrikshasana (tree). Notice the difference in balance between left and right.
Standing Flow Series. *Trikonasana* **(triangle)** to *Parshvakonasana* **(triangle II)** to *Parshvottanasana* **(angle).** Take only one side at a time. Feel the effects of left versus right or stronger versus weaker side. Are you feeling warm on one side? Off balance on the other?

Practice off the Mat

To find the pleasure in yoga as well as in life, focus on what you're doing, one thing at a time.

Wise Words

A posture isn't a posture unless you're breathing through it and thus connecting with it.

You can't measure the quality of your yoga practice on the depth of your forward bend or the flexibility of your hamstrings. It's not about how your postures look, but how they *feel*.

Notes

While we practice, keep in mind that combining the breath and the movement helps free the mind for a deeper awareness of the moment.

Keep your lines of energy long. Then lengthen those lines by filling your being with light, air and intention.

In every aspect of your life, it is important to find the balance between hurting and helping, pushing and pulling, and doing and non-doing.

When a posture becomes effortless, it becomes an opportunity to practice meditation.

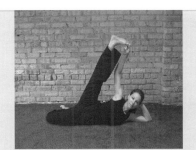

Serpent

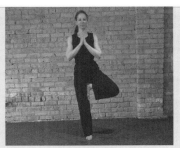

Vrikshasana
tree

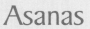

Asanas

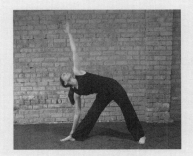

Trikonasana
triangle

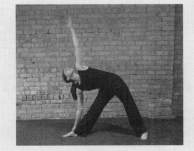

Standing flow Series
Parshvakonasana
triangle II

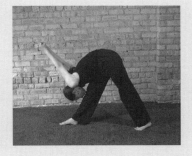

Parshvottanasana
angle

Chapter Two

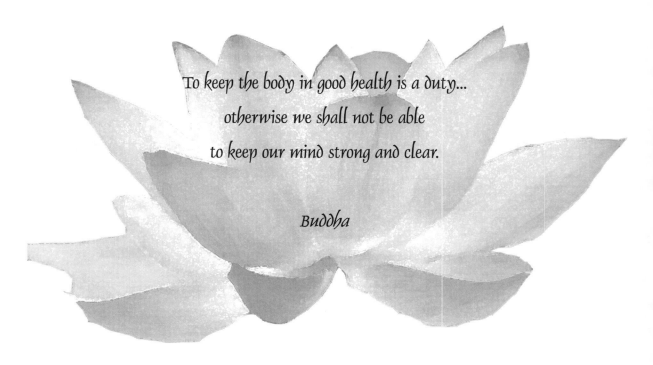

To keep the body in good health is a duty...

otherwise we shall not be able

to keep our mind strong and clear.

Buddha

Intermediate Breathing Lessons

This section is shaped to further your practice and teaching for complete breathing. At the core, these are the tools for better health, better living, and better awareness of your life. The teacher of peace will need these tools, so use them carefully.

In all of the lessons, being able to establish the complete diaphragmatic breath is key. If the breath is shallow or uneven, these exercises will be non-productive and may even cause dizziness or lightheadedness.

Minding the breath is a decision to live in this very moment — the only thing we can really be sure of.

And so we embark on the training for a yogic life.

Notes

2 to 1 Breathing

Intention: To live a more relaxed life even during stressful times; to feel the power of the exhalation during *asana.*
Approximate Length: 3-5 minutes

Lie in *shavasana.* Gently leave your past and your future. Keep your attention in the now, the feeling of your body on the ground, the sound of my voice, the awareness of your breath. If your attention is focused, then your mind is also focused.

Let the breathing be free and easy, and establish your diaphragmatic breath. Observe your abdomen rise and fall.

When we feel stress either in body or mind, our breathing becomes quite shallow and we breathe from the chest. This causes our inhalation to be longer than our exhalation, which in turn causes added toxins and tensions to build up — making us vulnerable to more anxiety.

The simple process of 2 to 1 breathing lengthens our exhale, so it's twice as long as our inhale. This quickly calms us down, releases mental tensions, and induces a natural state of relaxation.

Let's try this right now by gently slowing down the exhalation until we're exhaling to a mental count of four and inhaling to a count of two. Pull in the abdomen slightly to get a longer exhalation. Don't force the breath on either the in-breath or out-breath, we're simply changing the rhythm of breath. (Pause 1-3 minutes.)

Return to normal diaphragmatic breathing.

We're going to use this 2 to 1 breath in many of our *asanas* today so it's important to pay attention to the quality and length of your breathing.

Asanas for Deepening

Practice any standing or seated forward bend such as ***Parshvottanasana* (angle)** and ***Baddha Konasana* (butterfly)** using 2 to 1 breathing. Observe how the torso moves and loosens with each exhale, increasing your level of patience and mental clarity.
Woodchopper. "Chop" the imaginary wood between your legs with a long exhale.

Practice off the Mat

When you know the technique of exhaling as long or longer than you inhale, it helps to release stress, allowing you to act instead of react.

Counting the length of breath at any time during your day, is a useful method of practicing *dharana* (concentration).

Wise Words

Each breath is like an ocean wave swelling and contracting.

Notice when you get distracted, it shows up in your breathing.

Continually challenge yourself to stay mindful.

Notes

Asanas

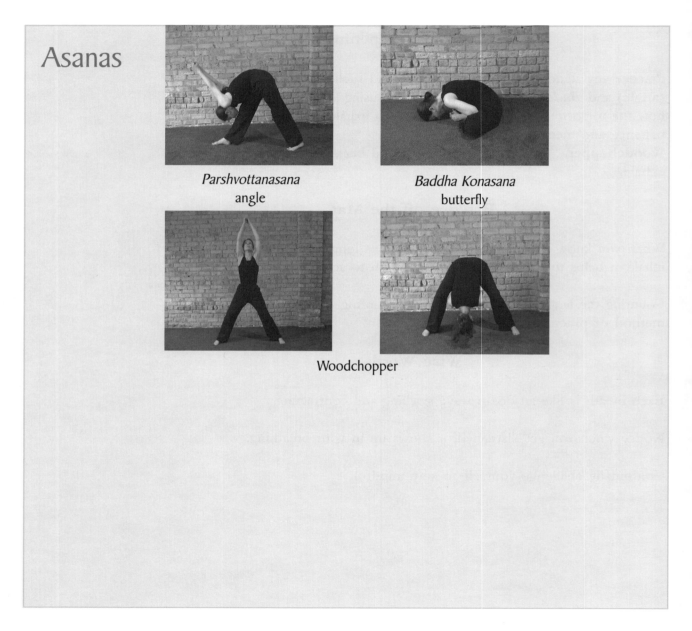

Parshvottanasana
angle

Baddha Konasana
butterfly

Woodchopper

3-Part Exhalation

Intention: To enhance exhalation and stimulate a deepening of inhalation. Beneficial for those with built-up tension.
Approximate Length: 3-4 minutes

Today we're going to consciously alter our breathing pattern so we can directly experience how this changes our thinking patterns.

We will be lengthening the exhalation by dividing it into 3 equal parts — pausing briefly between each consecutive exhalation.

This produces a longer exhalation than you might normally take. The 3-part exhale is useful if you have trouble falling asleep, getting rid of anxiety and for those times when you have a build-up of tension, common during menstruation and menopause.

Begin by taking a normal breath in and then divide your exhalation into three equal parts so you are emptying the breath from the top of the torso to the bottom — from throat center to pubic bone.

Like this: inhale completely, then exhale from the throat to the heart — pause, exhale from the heart to the navel — pause, exhale from the navel to the pubic bone — pause, then inhale completely again. Let each part of the exhalation be of equal length. The pauses between the sections of exhalation should feel like a moment of hesitation rather than a feeling of holding the breath.

Take a couple of normal breaths in and out, then repeat the 3-part exhalation.

You may imagine each exhalation as a soft leaf flowing slowly down to earth, gently touching the tree branches at each pause until it reaches the ground.

Or visualize yourself walking down a tall staircase exhaling as you step down, pausing at each step then descending further.

Or you may just want to visualize the breath moving from the throat to heart center, heart center to navel center, navel center to pubic bone. Try about 10 breath cycles, then relax.

Asanas for Deepening

Seated Twists: **Noose Twist or** *Marichyasana* **(half spinal twist)**. Utilize 3-part exhale to twist into the pose.
Prasarita Padottanasana **(spread leg forward bend)**. Use a 3-part exhale to take the pose. Note how applying a relaxed breath helps to relax the pose itself. Inhale and fill your posture with breath.
Setu Bandha Sarvangasana **(bridge)**. Release the pose with a 3-part exhale, feeling each section of vertebrae touch the earth.

Practice off the Mat

Consider your time on the mat a way to sweep through your energy field, erasing both mental and physical debris. Like weeding your garden, you're cleansing and creating more space for growth. Feel the lightness as you allow the mindfulness of yoga practice to lift the weight of your worries from your consciousness.

Wise Words

A focused mind directs *prana*.

If we are filled with toxins, tensions and closed-down body parts, how will we find room to store *prana*?

Stretch the breath as long as you can.

Asanas

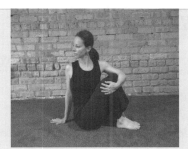

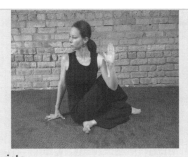

Seated Twists

Noose Twist

Marichyasana

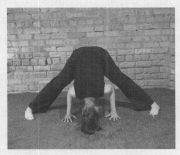

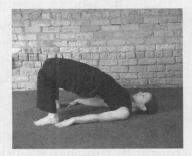

Prasarita Padottanasana
spread leg forward bend

Setu Bandha Sarvangasana
bridge

Ujjayi **Breath**

Intention: To bring a deeper awareness of the postures by internalizing attention.

Approximate Length: 3-4 minutes

Today we are going to learn *ujjayi* breath. Unlike regular diaphragmatic breathing, where the throat is relaxed and the breath is silent, *ujjayi* uses an audible vibration with some purposeful tension.

This type of breathing during *asana* or some *pranayamas* soothes the nerves and calms the mind. The sound naturally draws attention to the breath and internalizes focus. It also helps develop awareness of the subtle body and psychic sensitivity.

Plus, using *ujjayi* during *asana* practice is an excellent preparation for meditation.

Ujjayi requires breathing against the resistance of a constricted glottis — the aperture in the throat that opens and closes to hold the breath. It is located just behind the Adam's apple. The closing of the glottis is what allows pressure to build up before a cough and closes when you hold liquid in your mouth to gargle.

Ujjayi has a very distinctive sound. It sounds a little like the ocean waves. (Demonstrate the breath, coming around for each student to hear).

The breath is deeper than normal. The easiest way to deepen the breath is simply to expand the abdomen fully during inhalation and to contract it completely during exhalation.

To learn this, whisper "ha" with the mouth open on the exhale, and whisper "ah" on the inhale. Then gradually close the mouth. You should begin to feel the glottis.

You'll hear a short pause in the sound of *ujjayi* after inhalation and exhalation, but don't allow a pause in the breathing itself. Each inhale flows into the next exhale.

Be attentive to the soothing effects on the mind and the nervous system. We're going to be working with *ujjayi* through most of our *asana* practice.

Asanas for Deepening

Ujjayi leads to a deeper awareness of the posture by internalizing the attention.

Padmasana **(lotus)**/or **Easy Pose**. Inhale *ujjayi,* feel the breath move up the spine and mentally repeat the mantra *so*. Then as you exhale, feel the breath move down the spine, and mentally repeat *ham*.
Lunge Series. Work with long, deep *ujjayi* breaths in lunge, lunge with heel to hip and lunge with elbows on the ground toward the inside of the front foot.

Practice off the Mat

When possible, let life unfold organically, like a yoga pose. It doesn't mean dominating the situation or the body.

As with each breath, experience the newness of now.

Wise Words

Ujjayi helps promote internalization of the senses.

Ujjayi is a combination of two Sanskrit words, *ud* meaning up and *jayi,* meaning victory.

Be patient with yourself if you forget *ujjayi* after only a few breaths. Continued practice will allow you to keep track of both the posture and the breath.

Notes

59

Asanas

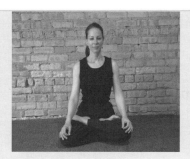

Padmasana
lotus

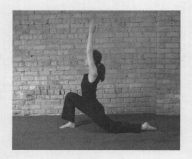

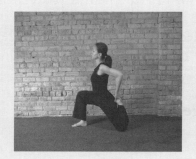

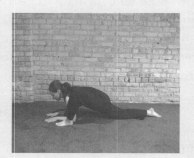

Lunge Series

Nadi Shodhana

Intention: To teach alternate nostril breathing and its benefits.
Approximate Length: 8-10 minutes

Can be practiced at the beginning, middle or end of class.

In *pranayama* or yoga breathing exercises, we seek to control *prana* — the vital energy within us. There are over 72,000 *nadis* or subtle energy channels in our body where *prana* moves. If the *nadis* are blocked, *prana* can't move freely through the body, consciousness is inhibited and it's difficult to attain meaning from our daily lives.

This can result in all the manifestations of suffering: distraction, dullness, anger, fear, anxiety. But as the *nadis* are purified — cleansed — *prana* can travel freely and consciousness is awakened.

Nadi shodhana is a breathing exercise that helps purify the *nadis*, focusing most directly on the two main *nadis*, the *pingala* and the *ida*. *Pingala* ends at the right nostril; *ida* ends at the left.

Pingala — the right nostril, embodies the sun and has a heating effect on the body. It's linked to left brain function and is associated with active external energy, intellectual pursuits and rational reasoning. When this nostril is open, it's good for taking a math test, making a sales presentation, even digesting food.

Ida — the left nostril, represents the moon and has a cooling effect on the body. This is linked to internal energy and the right side of the brain. It's connected to imagination, intuitive thinking and subjective decisions. When this nostril is open, it's great for creative thinking, poetry writing, listening to music or painting.

In *nadi shodhana*, we alternate our breath between the right and left nostrils seeking to balance the energies of the sun and the moon. When the *nadis* are cleared and energies are balanced, *prana* can flow more smoothly.

Notes

Let's try one round together. Sit in a comfortable seated position, head, neck and trunk in alignment. Breathe into each nostril separately to see which one is flowing more smoothly. Chances are, you will have an active nostril and a passive nostril. Begin your practice on your active side. Establish a natural diaphragmatic breath.

• Bring the right hand to the nose, folding the index finger and middle finger so that the right thumb can be used to close the right nostril and the right ring finger can be used to close the left nostril. Inhale through the nostrils.
• Close the passive nostril and exhale through the active nostril.
• Inhale through the active nostril slowly and completely.
• At the end of inhalation, close the active nostril and exhale and inhale through the passive nostril slowly and completely.
• Repeat this cycle of exhaling and inhaling two more times.
• At the end of the final inhalation on the passive nostril, exhale through both nostrils and take three very deep breaths. This completes one round.

To sum up one round of *nadi shodhana:*
1. Exhale Active
2. Inhale Active
3. Exhale Passive
4. Inhale Passive
5. Exhale Active
6. Inhale Active
7. Exhale Passive
8. Inhale Passive
9. Exhale Active
10. Inhale Active
11. Exhale Passive
12. Inhale Passive

Asanas for Deepening

Each nostril relates to different physiological aspects of our being.

After practicing a series of deep backbends, such as **Setu Bandha Sarvangasana (bridge), Bhujangasana (cobra)** or **Ustrasana (camel)**, typically very stimulating, check to see if the right nostril is active. Do the same for passive hold poses such as seated forward bends, like **Garland** or **Child's Pose**. Check to see if the left nostril is more open.

Finally, check the nostrils at the end of class. Our aim is to have both nostrils flowing smoothly and openly so *sushumna* is activated, the central main *nadi* that runs along the spine and ends at the crown *chakra*.

Practice off the Mat

Practice *nadi shodhana* anytime you need to quiet and calm the mind. Alternate nostril breathing is recommended twice a day. Try it once and you'll feel the effects immediately.

I knew a student who, during a heated business meeting excused herself to go the ladies room to practice *nadi shodhana*. She came back feeling refreshed, clear and courageous enough to tackle the rest of the meeting.

Alternate nostril breathing is also beneficial for insomnia and a common remedy for headaches.

Notes

Notes

Wise Words

Once you affirm the fact that you're exactly where you want to be, doing exactly what you want to be doing at this moment, you'll be amazed at how much energy is suddenly within you.

Listen to the sound of your breath, feel it in every cell, and imagine that the breath is stretching you.

The more awakened the *pranic* field, the more energetic we feel.

Sense the air as it empties and fills the lungs. Feel how the breath cleanses and nourishes.

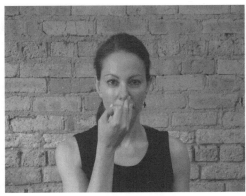

Pingala
breathing right nostril

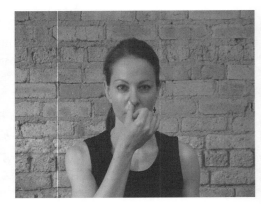

Ida
breathing left nostril

Asanas

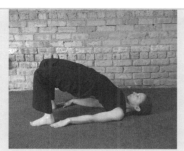

Setu Bandha Sarvangasana
bridge

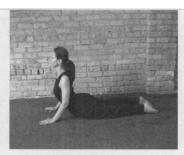

Bhujangasana
cobra

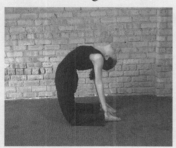

Ustrasana
camel

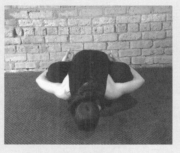

Garland

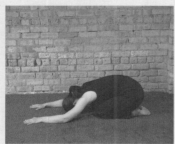

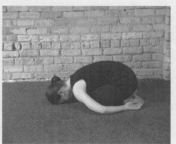

Child's Pose Variations

65

Chapter Three

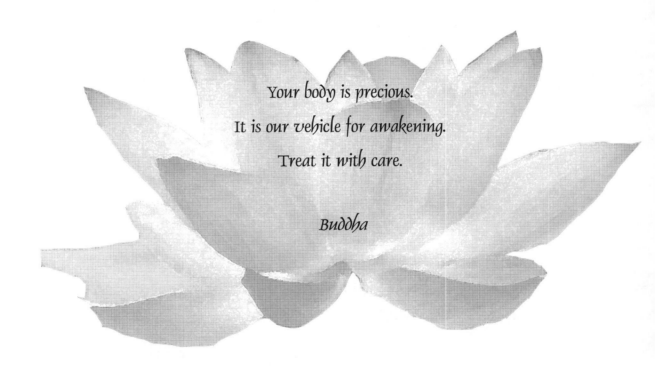

Your body is precious.

It is our vehicle for awakening.

Treat it with care.

Buddha

Asana

Asana, the third limb along the Royal Path, is very powerful practice. Simply by engaging our own internal intelligence, we can more clearly advance the practice of healing by penetrating deep layers of consciousness.

Open your mind to creativity within your postures. If you find, for instance, there's a whole new feeling in *trikonasana* when you turn your arm this way or that, share it with your students and fellow teachers. The practice and teaching becomes more inspiring, organic and alive the deeper you delve into your own self-discovery process.

Guide the way.

Feet

Intention: To practice feeling the body's foundation and utilizing earth energy through it.
Approximate Length: 2-3 minutes

Begin the class in *tadasana* or mountain pose.

Do you know how important your feet are? The average person takes 10,000 steps a day. The feet are our foundation. If our foundation is weak, problems may arise in the rest of the body. Many aches and pains from the ankles to the knees, the back, even the shoulders can be traced to issues in the feet.

In all of the standing poses, the part of the body that touches the ground forms the foundation. If the foundation of a house is out of alignment, the walls won't be straight and may crack. In *asana* practice, if the feet are misaligned or the body weight is off center on the feet, it will be very difficult to have a tall, spacious and centered pose.

Ideally, the weight of your body should be evenly distributed between the outer and inner foot, and between the heel and ball of the foot.

As you stand, become aware of the four corners of the foot: the ball of the big toe, the ball of the little toe, the inner heel and the outer heel.

If the inner foot feels heavy, the arch may be collapsing. If the outer foot is heavy, the arch of the foot may be high, but the base of the big toe may be lifting and the outer ankle could feel strain. Take a moment to check your foundation.

To make a strong, well-balanced foundation, the arch should feel lifted and light, while the inner heel and ball of your big toe stay grounded.

Let's use this foundation consciousness in our postures today.

Asanas for Deepening

Tadasana **(mountain pose)**. Spread the toes and snuggle the soles of the feet to the ground. Let the weight of the body merge downward. Feel the openings rise up to the crown. The weight of the body goes down, inner feeling rises up.

In all standing poses from *Trikonasana* **(triangle)** to any variation of *Virabhadrasana* **(warrior)** notice the position of feet and feel the lightening bolt of energy from the ground coming in through the soles. *Vrikshasana* **(tree)**. Establish the balanced action of your right arch, ankle, and toes in *Tadasana* **(mountain)**. Much of the work is done before the left foot is lifted off the ground. First, imagine a root extending from each of the four corners of the right foot down into the earth. From that root system, lift up from the arch of the foot through the leg to the pelvic floor and from the pelvic floor through the spine to the crown of the head. Finally, lift the left foot and place it on the right leg.

Sit on toes. Toes are curled under toward the floor.

Baddha Konasana **(butterfly).** Take a forward bend with forehead aimed toward toes. According to ancient teachings, the feet are symbols of humility and peace. Bringing the head, the seat of the ego, and the feet together help cultivate more humble and introspective characteristics within our personality.

Tennis Ball Massage. While standing, roll a tennis ball under the soles of feet. This is especially effective for sensitive soles (souls!).

Practice off the Mat

Keep your foundation healthy by walking barefoot whenever you can, spreading your toes frequently throughout the day and wearing comfortable shoes.

Notes

Reflexology speculates that by massaging the nerves in the feet, we can stimulate corresponding body parts. For instance, the big toe is said to relate to all glands and organs within the entire head.

Wise Words

Practice breathing easily in all standing poses, securing your foundation.

Feel earth energy coming in through the feet, up the legs, and settle into the pelvic floor. From there, make the pose more open and spacious by using the pelvic floor energy and spreading it through the rest of the body.

Keep the feet active through your practice, the balls of the feet extending forward and the toes spread. Use as much of your feet as you can.

If toes overlap, separate your toes with your fingers.

Asanas

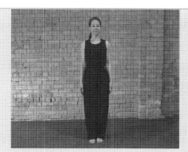

Tadasana
mountain

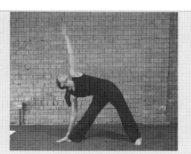

Trikonasana
triangle

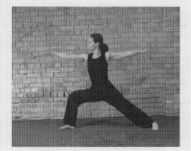

Virabhadrasana II
warrior II

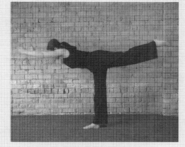

Virabhadrasana III
warrior III

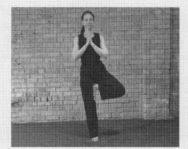

Vrikshasana
tree

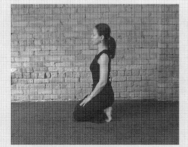

Sitting on Toes

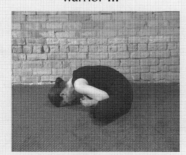

Baddha Konasana
butterfly

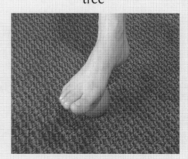

Tennis Ball Massage

Forward Bends

Intention: To develop a quiet and patient mind through the settling effects of forward bends.
Approximate Length: 2 minutes

If backbends are stimulating and exhilarating, then forward bends are just the opposite — they are quieting and settling. They bring us inward, making them very effective counterposes to the more vigorous backbends. And because they are an excellent antidote for anxiety, they require and develop an infinite amount of patience, perseverance and humility.

Physically they stretch and lengthen the spine, the muscles of the lower back, the pelvis and legs. The upper back, kidneys and adrenal glands are stretched and stimulated. They are excellent for relieving a mild backache.

The influences of the mind are observed throughout our entire practice, but forward bends, especially sustained forward bends, are important for understanding that yoga takes a more mental than physical effort.

When you hold a forward bend, you begin to see all the melodramas inside your head. Test your patience and see if you can wait out those little mind performances until they drop away completely.

Be sure to balance the forward bend sequences with backbends and twists.

Asanas for Deepening

Paschimottanasana **(posterior stretch)**. Ideal *asana* to examine the ebb and flow of mind. Emphasize the length of the front torso and deepen slowly with the breath, rather than folding completely to your edge.

Uttanasasa (**standing forward bend**). Continue letting go over and over using the power of the breath.

Child's Pose. Bring hands to the feet with palms up. Every other breath hum your exhalation.

Practice off the Mat

Forward bends help us remember what Buddhists call the Middle Way: not too much, not too little. Try to bring this philosophy into your daily life. For instance, when making a decision, whether it's what to eat for lunch or how to act toward an unfavorable colleague, practice the Middle Way.

Honor your boundaries in life, but expect them to expand. Have fun and faith!

Wise Words

Paschimottanasana has been labeled "the stretch of the west." It describes the ancient ritual of yogis facing the sunrise as they practiced. Yogis were literally stretching the west side or back side of the body as they bent toward the sun.

Recognizing what is true for you can be difficult if you want to be at a place you aren't ready for.

Explore any negative mental patterns you're bringing to the *asana* like an urge to push or a tendency to let the mind wander.

Notes

Asanas

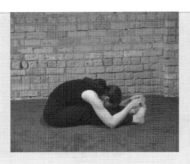

Paschimottanasana
Posterior Stretch

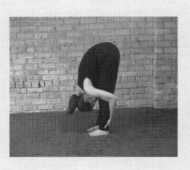

Uttanasana
standing forward bend

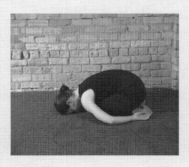

Child's Pose

Backbends

Intention: To understand the physiological aspects of backbends.
Approximate Length: 2-3 minutes

Yoga is defined as the restraint of the fluctuations of the mind. Our practice is intended to reduce these fluctuations in the frontal lobe of the brain, the part that is most involved in conscious thought.

Our time on the mat is spent moving from the familiar to the somewhat obscure, from the front part of the brain to the back of the brain, from the front of our bodies — the known, to the back of our bodies — the unknown.

Today were going to bring this awareness into our backbends. Backbending *asanas* bolster a sense of openness, confidence and bravery. They open the chest, abdominal organs, and pelvic region — basically the whole front side of the body.

Yoga is about oneness and integration of body-mind-spirit. So when there are areas in the body — front, back or side — that are closed down, it makes us feel separate and limits energy flow. This can cause mild depression, fear and weakness.

The physical aspects of backbending work counter to these emotions because they improve circulation along the spine, helping to relieve depression and other symptoms of feeling "closed off." Ultimately they leave us feeling refreshed and alive.

Be sure to balance backbends with forward bends, twists and neutralizing poses like child's pose.

Asanas for Deepening

Before beginning the backend, lengthen the pose first, then go for depth. Depth without length creates constriction.

Notes

Even and steady breathing with a focus on completing the exhalation inhibits overstimulation of your sympathetic nervous system. This makes for a calmer pose.

Practice a series of *asanas* to work up to ***Chakrasana* (wheel)**, such as **Standing Backbend,** *Bhujangasana* **(cobra)** unsupported and supported, *Ustrasana* **(camel),** *Urdhva Mukha Shvanasana* **(updog),** *Dhanurasana* **(bow), Inverted Table** and *Setu Bandha Sarvangasana* **(bridge)**.

Practice off the Mat

Simple backbends such as unsupported cobra and bridge are highly recommend *asanas* for anyone with breathing difficulties such as asthma. They can be exhilarating, creating openings in the chest, ribs and collarbone areas, consequently allowing inhalation to flow more freely. They are also beneficial for times in the day when you're feeling sluggish and need a quick pick-me-up-*asana*.

Wise Words

The real power of backbends is subtle. They work on the nervous system, which is one reason why they're helpful in easing mild depression.

Backbends are a bit mysterious and provocative because they engage a part of the body we literally can't see.

Let the posture be your tool so you can hold more energy, more light. Make room for your spirit to be free.

Asanas

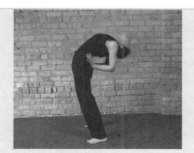

Standing Backbend

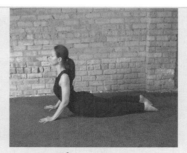

Bhujangasana
supported cobra

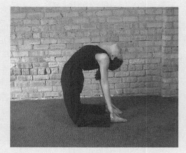

Ustrasana
camel

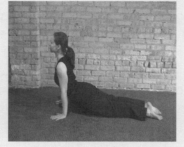

Urdhva Mukha Shvanasana
updog

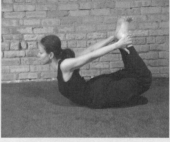

Dhanurasana
bow

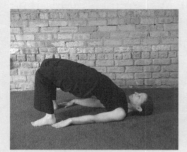

Setu Bandha Sarvangasa
bridge

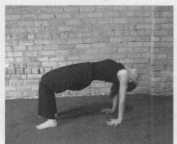

Inverted Table

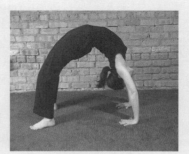

Chakrasana
wheel

Twists

Intention: To learn to twist properly so that body and mind receive a "squeeze and release" effect.
Approximate Length: 3-4 minutes

Today our focus will be on twists. The twist is the great equalizer: if you're tired they pick you up, if you're anxious they help calm you down.

The virtue of the twist is to wring out the body and assist in releasing tension. When we release the twisting — the wringing out action — and the muscles relax again, those areas that were involved in the twist become flooded with nutrients and fresh blood.

Twists tone and cleanse your organs, release and strengthen the muscles of your spine and neck, and allow you to open and strengthen your shoulder joints. As the torso rotates, the kidneys and abdominal organs are activated and exercised. This improves digestion and removes sluggishness.

And, since every nerve begins in the spinal cord, every part of the body rejuvenates, heals and becomes more vital. We are then more comfortable in our bodies and more inspired with lifeforce.

Let's discuss the physical principles of the twist by taking a simple seated twist in easy pose, pelvis in neutral.

Put your awareness at the crown of your head — open the crown so the chest, neck and head are lifted. Then elongate and align the spine by pressing both sit bones downward into the floor. Bring your left hand to your right knee and right hand behind you. Inhale and lift, exhale and gently rotate to the right from the base of the spine up into the low back, waist, shoulder blades and finally neck.

With every breath, continue to lengthen the spine, creating space in the vertebrae, making for a deeper and safer experience.

These principles will be included in all of the twists we'll be practicing today.

Remember to balance your twist practice with forward and backward bends.

Asanas for Deepening

Reclining Twist. Allow the rib cage to release and your feet and knees to settle to the earth.

Seated Twists: Noose Twist, *Marichyasana* **(half spinal twist).**

Garudasana **(eagle).** Since most twists focus on the torso, this twist benefits both legs and arms.

Parivrtta Trikonasana **(revolved triangle).** Twist from the base of the spine and continue to twist to the crown.

Runner's Lunge Twist with *Namaste* **Hands**

Practice off the Mat

If you spend a lot of time in a chair, remember to take several "twist" breaks. Bring your knees to one side of the seat, hands to the arm you are twisting toward or to the back of the chair, extend upwards on your inhale and on your exhale, gently twist to the side your knees are facing.

Notes

Wise Words

Twists keep *avidya*, spiritual tunnel vision, out of our lives. By staying present with everything both around us and in back of us, we keep our inner vision clear and unobstructed by illusion.

Twists allow us to stay present during all of life's changes.

Before you begin the actual twisting movement, get as long as you can by pressing downward and reaching upward.

Feel the spine come to life.

Asanas

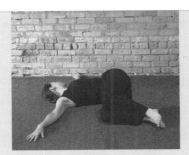

Reclining Twist

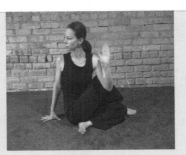

Marichyasana
half spinal twist

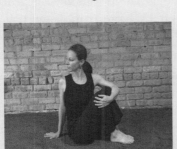

Noose Twist

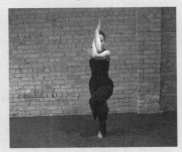

Garudasana
eagle

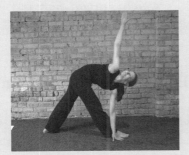

Parivrtta Trikonasana
revolved triangle

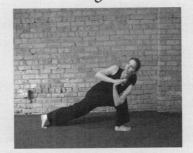

Runner's Lunge Twist
with *Namaste* Hands

Headstand

Intention: To enjoy the benefits of the "king of *asana*."
Approximate Length: 2-3 minutes

Shirshasana or headstand is known as the king of *asana* because it has legendary benefits ranging from increasing vitality, helping with insomnia, improving concentration and toning the glandular system.

However, accomplishing headstand can be a significantly challenging achievement. Some of us have trouble with it because either we don't have enough strength and flexibility in our shoulders and hamstrings or we have weak lower backs and abdominal muscles. Fortunately, there are a number of preparatory *asanas* that address these problems.

But, a third hurdle may be the most overlooked — headstand requires overcoming the anxiety and fear of turning upside down and the possibility of falling. For those of you who find yourself in this category, we'll use the wall for support.

Contraindications for practicing headstand include high blood pressure, heart problems, cervical spine injuries, detached retina, glaucoma, osteoporosis, neck injuries, excess weight, pregnancy and menstruation.

Let's begin the headstand with some postures that lay the groundwork for the king of a*sana*.

Asanas for Headstand Preparation

Some schools of yoga counter headstand with tadasana, while others follow with child's pose. Trust your inner teacher and stay connected with what feels best for you. Be sure to practice some or all of the following preparatory postures before demonstrating headstand.

Reclining Hamstring Stretch.   Opens hips and hamstrings.
Bhujangasana **(unsupported cobra)**.   Develops low back muscles.
Dolphin.   The classic pose for headstand preparation. Develops strength and flexibility in the shoulders, and strengthens the abdominal and back muscles.
Fire Series (leg lifts). Strengthens navel center.
Shoulder Stretches: arm swings, cow's face arms, eagle arms
Setu Bandha Sarvangasana **(bridge).**   Hands interlaced beneath spine, tops of shoulders rolled under, shoulder blades moving toward tailbone: opens entire upper chest, stretches spine.
Halasana **(plow)**
Sarvangasana **(shoulderstand)**
Matsyasana **(fish)**

Practice off the Mat

Keep thoughts positive.   Allow yourself to be guided from within.

Notice the confidence and inner strength that's revealed when headstand is practiced.

Headstand stimulates the crown *chakra*, our connection to divine spirit.

Wise Words

If balance changes as you take your legs slowly up into headstand, stop moving until you gain equilibrium.

Moment-to-moment awareness is the secret to balance.

Stretch your torso and soles of the feet up toward the sky.

Notes

Notes

Further deepen your headstand by adding *ujjayi* breath. *Ujjayi* is effortless in inversions as the throat is already compressed.

If you can remain in headstand for just three minutes, the blood will drain to the heart and tissue fluids will flow more efficiently into the veins and lymph channels of the lower extremities.

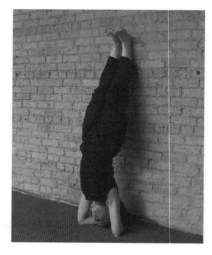

Shirshasana
headstand

Asanas

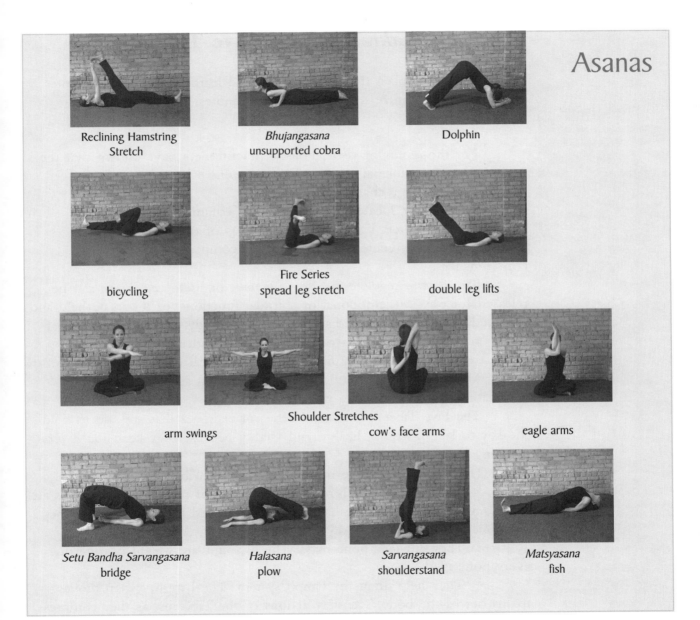

Reclining Hamstring
Stretch

Bhujangasana
unsupported cobra

Dolphin

bicycling

Fire Series
spread leg stretch

double leg lifts

Shoulder Stretches

arm swings

cow's face arms

eagle arms

Setu Bandha Sarvangasana
bridge

Halasana
plow

Sarvangasana
shoulderstand

Matsyasana
fish

Chakras and the Five Tibetans

Intention: To explain the *chakra* system and learn the Five Tibetan rites.
Approximate Length: Approximately 30 minutes (includes the Five Tibetans practice)

For thousands of years, holistic practitioners have known that the body has seven principal energy centers: *chakras* where the *nadis,* the body's subtle energy channels, intersect.

The *chakras*, located along the spinal column, are considered transformation centers linked to specific areas of the body and mind. These seven energy centers form the major components of our consciousness.

The *chakras* regulate the flow of *prana* or lifeforce. *Prana* can be released for physical, emotional or spiritual functions, or it can be held and ultimately blocked, causing disruptions in the body. An accumulation of toxins in the internal organs can also interfere with the flow of *prana*. When this happens, we may manifest psychological or somatic illnesses.

Many of these disharmonies can be treated successfully by readjusting and harmonizing the *chakras*.

The Five Tibetan rites are a series of exercises that are said to hold the key to lasting youth, health, and vitality because they keep the *chakras* spinning and balanced.

Here are some of the benefits of the Five Tibetans:

• They balance the hormones. When all of the endocrine glands are functioning in harmony, we have more energy and more vitality. Balanced hormones also help with PMS and menopausal discomforts.

• They enhance bone mass. The Tibetans are weight bearing on every bone in the body.

• They help drain the lymph system. The lymph system moves toxins out of the body. The very actions of the Tibetans, as they compress and stretch the various organs, glands and muscles assist in draining the lymph system. The result — you flush toxins faster.

The quickest way to regain youth, health, and vitality is to get these energy centers spinning normally again. The Five Tibetans do just that.

It takes about 20 minutes to perform the full 21 repetitions of each of these rites. For beginners, it's suggested that you start with 3-5 repetitions a day for the first week and increase the number by 2 every week until you reach the full 21 repetitions. Today we'll do 5 repetitions of each.

Guide students through a brief warm-up such as slow moving Surya Namaskara (sun salutations) before introducing the Five Tibetans.

Rite 1 — Spinning
Stand in mountain pose with arms outstretched, horizontal to the floor. Slowly spin around clockwise until you become slightly dizzy.

Rite 2 — Leg Lifts
Lie flat on the floor, face up. Extend your arms along your sides and place the palms of your hands against the floor. Inhale and raise your head off the floor, tucking the chin against the chest.

As you do this, lift your legs and bring your legs straight up into a vertical position. If possible, let the legs extend back over the body, toward the head. Exhale, slowly lowering both the head and the legs, to the floor.

Rite 3 — Camel
Kneel on the floor. Place the hands against the lower back. On exhale bring the head and neck forward, tucking the chin against the chest. Then on inhale bring the head and neck backward, arching the spine and tucking

in the tailbone. As you arch, brace your arms and hands against the low back for support. After inhale, return to the original position, starting over again.

Rite 4 — Table Lifts

Sit on the floor with your legs straight out in front of you and your feet about 12 inches apart. Place the palms of your hands on the floor alongside the hips. Tuck the chin against the chest. Inhale, gently bring the head backward as far as it will go and at the same time, raise your body so that the knees bend, tracking straight ahead towards the top of the feet, while the arms remain straight. The trunk of the body will be in a straight line with the upper legs, horizontal to the floor. Tense every muscle in the body. Exhale and relax your muscles as you return to the original sitting position.

Rite 5 — Updog/Downdog

Lie face down. Place your palms on the floor beneath your shoulders, and turn the toes under. Inhale and lift your head, neck and chest so arms are perpendicular to the floor and the spine is arched, pelvis lifted so the body is in a sagging position and legs are off the ground (updog). Exhale bend at the hips, bring the body up into an inverted "V" and at the same time, bring the chin forward, tucking it against the chest (downdog).

Relax in *shavasana* for 5 minutes.

Practice off the Mat

Practice the Five Tibetans every day for a week. Notice a welcome increase in energy levels with vitality lasting through the day. Many people reduce or stop their coffee consumption completely. Avoid practicing the Five Tibetans 2-3 hours before bedtime.

Wise Words

The symptoms of old age and physical degeneration set in when the *chakras* slow down.

Chanting *om* vibrates and awakens all the *chakras*.

The *chakras* are like traffic circles with the *nadis* connecting to each *chakra*.

Notes

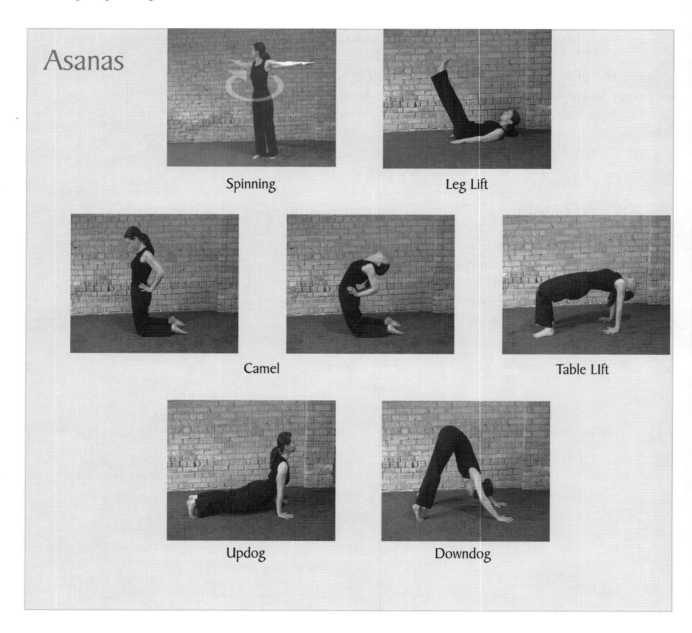

Asanas

Spinning

Leg Lift

Camel

Table LIft

Updog

Downdog

Asana and Acceptance

Intention: To define Patanjali's *asana*; to accept where we are in *asana* as in life.

Approximate Length: 2 minutes

In Patanjali's *Yoga Sutras*, the definition of *asana* is a pose that is both steady and comfortable. In this sense, the interpretation means to be fully present, to be exclusively alive to the now experience.

Learning to be present and participate in anything that is both steady and comfortable does not allow space for attachment such as self-judgement. When you live this way, you are practicing yoga — you are living thoroughly.

Many times in our practice, and in our lives, we respond from a place of judgment. "I can't do this posture" or "everyone else is more flexible than me" or the popular "this posture doesn't make any sense!"

Our practice is to not criticize yourself or anyone or anything for this next hour. If you do, just notice it, check to see if your judgment is placed on your emotions, your body or breath, and let it go.

Today if you find yourself forcing in *asana*, or in any other part of your life, ask yourself: is this in the spirit of the true practice of yoga?

When things are steady and comfortable, there is no forcing.

Asanas for Deepening

Teach postures that you and your class may find very challenging like **Virabhadrasana III (warrior III)**, *Hanumanasana* **(splits)** or *Tittibhasana* **(firefly)**. Break down the posture or use support such as a wall to demonstrate the potential ease and comfort anywhere in any *asana*. Everybody's "steady" and "comfortable" is different. *Asana* is not what it looks like, it's what it feels like. Teach students to find what feels right for each person.

Notes

Notes

Practice off the Mat

Take a look at your life. Notice areas that you'd like to be different or eliminated entirely, places that *do not* feel steady and comfortable. Can you make adjustments in your mindset as you do in your *asana*? Allow these areas in your life to flow through you so you can accept rather than agonize.

Feel yourself becoming sensitized and responsive. Put conscious passion into your life and sense the heightened perception.

Wise Words

Don't worry about what anyone thinks. The problem with acceptance is that it puts the power base outside of yourself.

Accept where you are in this moment without striving, without comparing or judging.

Go where it feels it best, where your energy flows best. Trust your ability to sense this.

If there's a place in your physical or emotional body that needs extra attention, invite that energy to surround that area of your life without judgment.

Asanas

Virabhadrasana III
warrior III

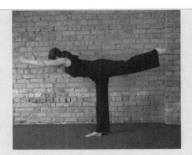

Tittibhasana
Firefly

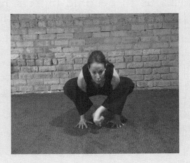

Asana and Peace

Intention: To learn that yoga practice can have a positive impact on peace.
Approximate Length: 2 minutes

Those of us who practice yoga receive many of the benefits of non-violence and a peaceful spirit.

Our *asana* practice alone has a positive impact on peace because it asks us to become more sensitive, more conscious and more aware of ourselves as bodies, as minds and as spirits. This awareness make us clearer and calmer, more awakened to truth and thus more able to handle life's endless challenges.

As we become more aware, we move away from forcing and controlling while we move toward letting the universe take care of many of our daily dilemmas. In turn, these changes influence the consciousness and actions of everyone we meet. The sensitivity we develop on our yoga mats affects everyone around us.

Slowly, yogi by yogi, we can shift the direction the world is taking.

Asanas for Deepening

Parrot (half squat, half lunge). The parrot symbolizes neutrality, the one who takes action without judgment, repeating what others say without attaching or analyzing.

Clam (easy pose with forward bend). Experience the wonder of being breathed. Ask yourself who is in control of this breathing. It happens 24 hours a day, every day for your whole life, without conscious effort. Now breathe awareness into your muscles. Don't let the breath get blocked anywhere along the way.

Peaceful Warrior Flow Series: *Virabhadrasana* **II to I to III.** Practice using the intuitive *feeling* of courage. Be bold. Feel the fortitude, the firmness, the determination it takes to practice the postures. Dare to confront the difficulties of life with a peaceful intent to face internal conflicts head on.

Practice off the Mat

The moment we start to force a situation, which can be especially true during times of impatience, we begin to lose awareness of our nervous system and the circumstance itself. Watch to see if you find yourself forcing or pushing. This will inevitably create struggle and discomfort. Breathe thoroughly and look for the place of peace in every situation.

Wise Words

Forcing the body past the point of resistance is an act of self-aggression and works counter to peace practice.

Spread peace wherever you go.

The surest way to make your own life happier is to do all you can to uplift the lives of others.

Notes

Asanas

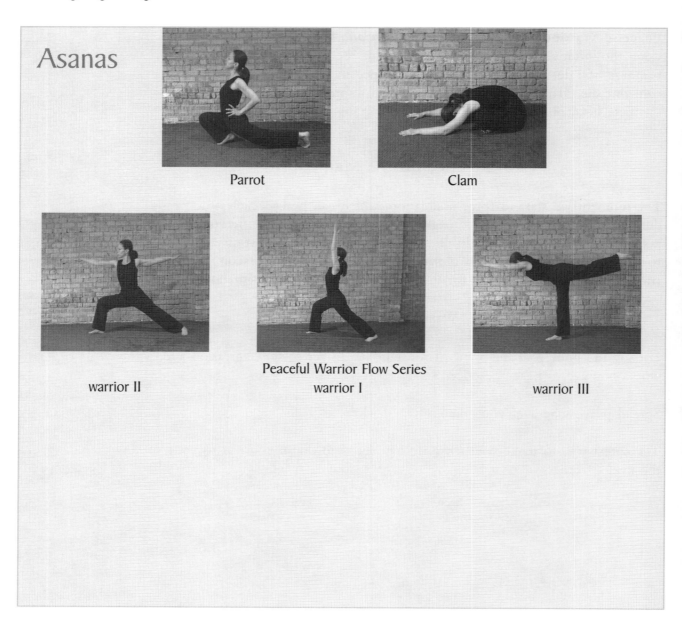

Parrot

Clam

warrior II

Peaceful Warrior Flow Series
warrior I

warrior III

Chapter Four

Thousands of candles can be lighted from a single candle
and the life of the candle will not be shortened.
Happiness never decreases by being shared.

Buddha

Prana

From my experience, a fundamental comprehension of *prana* can make or break one's yoga class experience.

The complexities of the *Hatha* Yoga journey are realized when we understand that the same lifeforce that illuminates me also illuminates you, the tree outside, the squirrel in that tree and the forest floor around the tree.

We not only get a clearer sense of how nature relates to our individual lifeforce, but how we are each but a wave in the ocean of life, *pranically* connected.

Holding on to *Prana*

Intention: To understand the discipline of maintaining *pranic* balance.
Approximate Length: 2-3 minutes

In order to better understand the holistic practice of yoga, it's important to know about this energy that we're made of.

Prana is a Sanskrit word meaning lifeforce or energy. It signifies the energy that flows through our *nadis,* our body's subtle energy channels.

The breath is the most significant way we bring lifeforce into our bodies. We also receive *prana* from food, sleep and emotion, such as love and happiness.

But if our emotions are disturbed, or our sleeping habits inadequate, our *prana* is scattered and our lifeforce is lost or wasted. To be strong and healthy, we have to learn how to keep our *prana* inside the body, direct it, and not let it seep out through disturbing circumstances.

We often have to step away from negative or draining situations in order to stay healthy. This discipline is vital for holding on to *prana,* allowing us to have enough left over to stay focused and balanced.

In *asana* practice, we train ourselves to watch for distractions and interruptions and notice when we wander off.

In today's practice, notice when the mind rambles and how long it takes to come back to the moment. This is how we begin to feel our lifeforce. We start to see that practice is changing us in some ways. Physically, we discover a few places where *prana* is blocked, such as the shoulders, neck or hips. Through mindfulness, we focus on the things we've been giving our energy to that we need to let go of.

When we first enter upon this awareness, we have officially begun to wake up!

Asanas for Deepening

Reclining Twists
Reclining Hamstring Stretch
Seated *Yoga Mudra*
***Surya Namaskara* (sun salutation)**. Practice uniting the body, mind and spirit in celebration of our existence and the vitality of the lifeforce within us.

Practice off the Mat

Become aware of how important attitude is in every aspect of your life. Attitude has the power to transform your experience of life itself. Live with intention.

Wise Words

If we are filled with toxins, tensions and closed-down body parts, we won't have room for *prana* to flow.

Stay centered by accepting whatever you are doing.

Prana follows thought.

Asanas

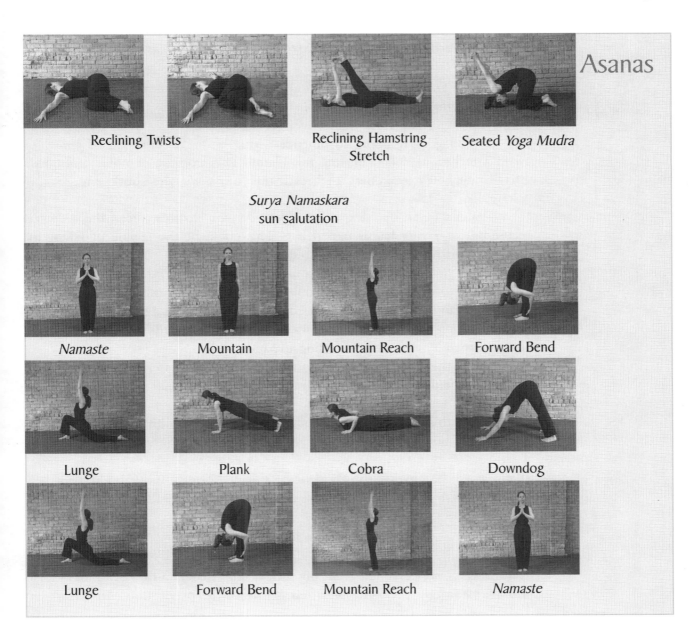

Reclining Twists

Reclining Hamstring
Stretch

Seated *Yoga Mudra*

Surya Namaskara
sun salutation

Namaste

Mountain

Mountain Reach

Forward Bend

Lunge

Plank

Cobra

Downdog

Lunge

Forward Bend

Mountain Reach

Namaste

Feeling the Flame

Intention: To get a direct sensation of *prana* as it relates to life experience.
Approximate Length: 3-5 minutes

Today we're going to practice getting a direct sensation of *prana* with a technique called Feeling the Flame. This exercise explores emotions that bring *pranic* awareness of breath into our *nadis*, the subtle energy channels.

Let's begin by lying in *shavasana*. As you do this, recall the sensation of a very happy experience. This could be the feeling of falling in love, the birth of a child, or a fabulous vacation.

As you see this experience in your mind's eye, inhale the experience and begin to spread your arms out slowly. With your inhale, visualize your breath expanding from your heart center. This is an expanding flame that moves your arms effortlessly upward toward your head. As your inner flame expands, your happy feeling expands with it.

Let the flame of happiness spread from the center of your heart, reaching out to the tips of your fingers, up to your head and down to your toes.

Do this 3 to 5 more times. Go slowly and rhythmically. As you open, your body fills with breath awareness and happiness all at once.

Please note: For many, the thought of warmth brings about body heat. *Prana* follows thought; be prepared to cool down!

Asanas for Deepening

With any *asana*, establish *pranic* intention. For instance in **Parshvot-tanasana** (angle), feel the *pranic* energy from the pelvic floor. In **Vira-**

bhadrasana I (warrior I), feel the *pranic* energy running from the back heel all the way up to the fingertips. In a seated forward bend, such as **Paschimottanasana (posterior stretch),** reach for your legs, ankle or toes as if you're reaching for someone or something you love.

Practice off the Mat

Whenever you're in need of the emotional power of your *prana,* you can get an instant vacation by creative visualization. Close your eyes and in your mind's eye, you could be on a sandy beach, a cabin in the woods, or in the moment you first fell in love.

Wise Words

During *asana,* focus more on what you're doing with your *prana* than your muscles. What happens to the breath when a posture is easy for you? What about when a posture is difficult? What happens to your mind?

During *asana,* imagine the muscles in a particular color, texture or emotion. Then change the color, texture or emotion and note how that affects your entire practice.

Notes

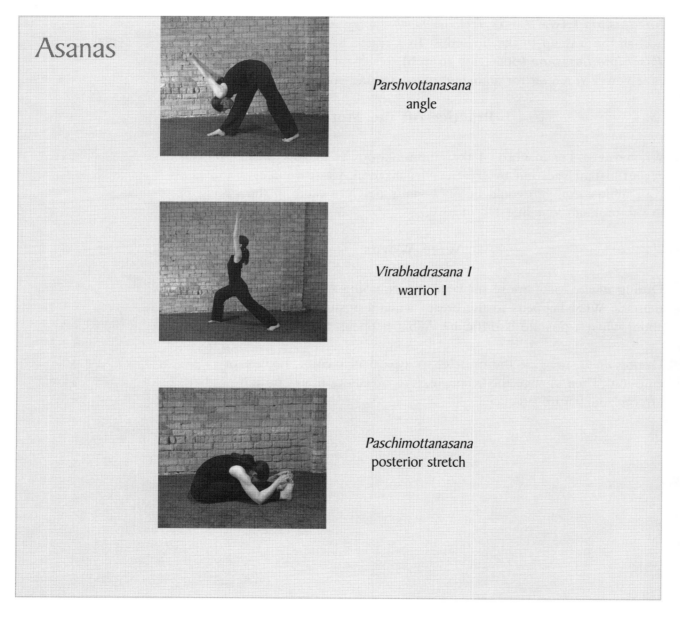

Asanas

Parshvottanasana
angle

Virabhadrasana I
warrior I

Paschimottanasana
posterior stretch

The Focused Mind and *Prana*

Intention: To understand how the mind affects *prana*.
Approximte Length: 2 minutes

Prana or lifeforce is the vital energy of the universe. The human body exists by the same *prana* that sustains every living thing around us, just as the ocean is represented by a single drop.

Prana can be increased and decreased at will and moved here and there where we may need it. The process of learning postures, breathing techniques and practicing meditation is to learn to consciously control and move *prana*.

When we deal with situational circumstances like managing stress, we can actually lose lifeforce. For instance, if we're worried about 10 different things we may have *prana* bursting out of us in 10 different directions.

If you're angry with someone or something right now, you're giving some of your available *prana*, your precious lifeforce, to that person or situation. This is draining to your energy and toxic to your system.

Learning to detach from negative situations is vital for keeping *prana* flowing. When we work with *prana* intelligence, we work with and through stress, negative situations and behaviors to create a quiet, calm, mindful mind.

Asanas for Deepening

Our *asana* practice gives us a system for identifying when, where and how we are losing or blocking off energy. As you go through your postures, you begin to notice where you're tight, weak, distracted or uncomfortable.

Ardha Chandrasana **(half moon)**. Focus on the supporting leg, moving energy into the pelvis and out into the limbs.
Kapotasana **(pigeon)**. Backbend and resting variations.

Practice off the Mat

Keep your *prana*. Try to limit your time and energy with those you may find toxic. These could be co-workers, relatives, even friends from whom you need to distance yourself.

Practice *Bhastrika* Breath (bellows) whenever you need a quick energy boost. Try 3 rounds of 11 breaths, drawing air in and out of the lungs very quickly. *Bhastrika* breath builds mastery of the energy flow in the body, energizing every cell, and awakening serpent power (*kundalini*).

Wise Words

To keep *prana* flowing, focus on the moment. The concentration of mindfulness helps us remember that we can't tune into our yoga practice and be absorbed in a personal drama at the same time.

After holding postures such as the seated twist, remember to feel the increased flow of energy through the spine.

A focused mind directs *prana*.

Asanas

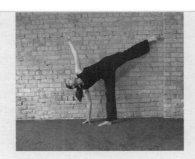

Ardha Chandrasana
half moon

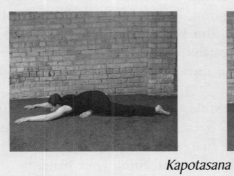 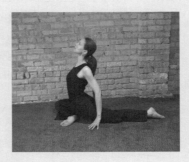

Kapotasana

resting pigeon   backbend pigeon

Storing *Prana*

Intention: To gain experiential knowledge of storing *prana*.
Approximate Length: 5-7 minutes with *prana* generating exercise

Most of us begin yoga to experience the physical benefits. But we stay because we begin to feel the esoteric benefits, many of which come from yoga's *pranic* power.

Prana is interwoven within the entire philosophy of *Hatha* Yoga and should be understood and acclimated within all of our yoga practices.

To illustrate this point, in ordinary breathing we absorb an adequate supply of *prana*. But by controlled and regulated breathing exercises we can elicit a greater supply so that we can store and use *prana* when we need it. We can then stockpile *prana* just as a storage battery can store electricity.

Today we'll work with a breathing exercise that stores *prana* in the solar plexus — the body's great central *prana* storehouse, as well the place that radiates strength and energy to all parts of the body.

Please lie down in *shavasana*. Bring your hands to the solar plexus and breathe rhythmically. After the rhythm is established, visualize how each inhalation draws in an expansive supply of *prana* or vital energy from the universal supply. This *prana* is taken in by the nervous system and stored in the solar plexus.

On each exhalation, feel how each breath radiates strength and energy to all parts of the body. Feel how the vital energy is distributed all over to every organ, every muscle, every bone, every vein, every cell, from the top of your head to the soles of your feet, invigorating, recharging and stimulating every nerve, sending energy and power through every layer of consciousness.

Envision in-rushing *prana* coming in through the lungs and flowing into the solar plexus. Then exhale and savor the lifeforce being sent to all parts of the system, out to the fingertips and down to the toes.

Asanas for Deepening

Agni Sara - **fanning.** Fans the flame of the solar plexus and distributes lifeforce. Helps open and work the abdominal muscles, intestines, ovaries, fallopian tubes, uterus, spleen, gall bladder, kidneys, diaphragm and lower back. In a standing position, bend forward and rest your hands just above your knees. Exhale completely, pulling your belly back toward the spine. Without inhaling, let the belly drop, pull it back in again, let it drop, pull it back in again. Repeat this process until you need to inhale. Repeat 2-3 times and feel the heat.
Navasana **(sitting boat).** Creates strength in the solar plexus.
Kapotanasa **(pigeon).** Stretches the solar plexus and opens the hips.

Practice off the Mat

Smile at any time during the day and notice the calming effect on the body and heart center.

Look outside. Contemplate how nature is never at rest. From the smallest blade of grass to the world's largest ocean, everything is alive with *pranic* vibration.

Wise Words

Use intention. Do you want to stretch the hamstrings? Calm an anxious mind? Make a decision? When inhaling universal energy and consequently allowing that energy to spread throughout the body, make a mental picture of what you want to produce.

Notes

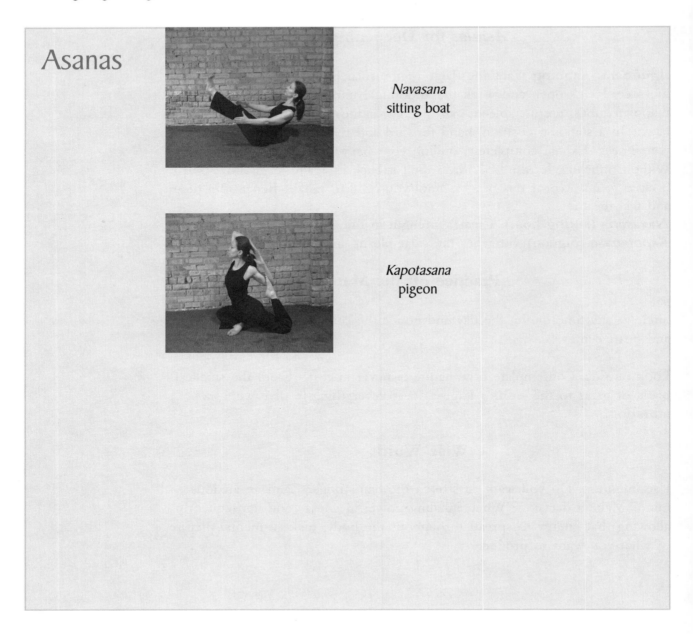

Asanas

Navasana
sitting boat

Kapotasana
pigeon

Chapter Five

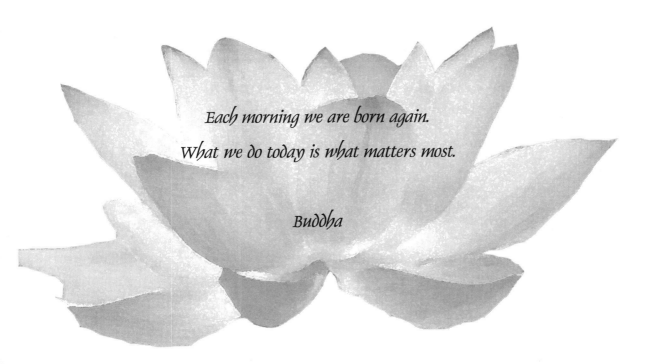

Each morning we are born again.

What we do today is what matters most.

Buddha

Pranayama

Our *Hatha* Yoga practices are designed to help unclog the *nadis,* the body's subtle energy channels, so that *prana* can flow freely and we can direct it toward more spiritual endeavors.

Pranayama, the fourth of the eight-limbed path of *Raja* Yoga is also referred to as the last of the so-called external limbs. Although sometimes taught completely separate from postures or neglectfully not at all, *asana* practice helps prepare us for more advanced *pranayama* exercises by reducing body tension, opening up the breathing anatomy, and bringing awareness to the flow of breath.

Asana, united with *pranayama* and rightful living, directly support the aspirant with his/her journey to enlightenment.

On this glorious path of liberation, we must visit all the stops along the road.

What is *Pranayama?*

Intention: To get a basic knowledge of the science and practice of *pranayama* and how it relates to the Royal Path.
Approximate Length: 2 minutes
Pranayama practice after relaxation: 5 minutes

Pranayama is the fourth limb of the eight-limbed Royal Path as taught by Patanjali. Many students know it as a variety of breathing practices.

The word itself is a combination of *prana,* or lifeforce, and *yama,* meaning control. The practice of *pranayama* is the science of breath that brings lifeforce under control.

Pranayama's purpose is to be an instrument that helps to control the thought waves of the mind. When we have controlled the breath and *prana,* we have controlled the mind. The act of inhalation is the process of uniting universal energy with the individual breath. Exhalation is the removal of toxins from the system.

A regular *pranayama* practice keeps the *nadis,* the body's subtle energy channels, in good health and prevents their decay.

Additionally, the physical practice of *pranayama* dynamically increases our lung capacity. We breathe 23,000 times per day, using 4500 gallons of air. With regular practice we can learn to deepen the breath and utilize up to 6000 gallons of air a day.

Today, after relaxation, we'll have a short *pranayama* practice using *Anuloma Krama.* This breath is a segmented inhalation that fills the torso with *prana* and expands our lung capacity.

Asanas for Deepening

Any practice that prepares the body for pranayama should stretch and strengthen the supporting anatomy around the lungs and diaphragm.

Thread the Needle. On hands and knees, thread left arm in back of right arm and draw left shoulder blade to the ground. Twist to the right. Repeat on the opposite side.

Standing Spread-legged Forward Bend with Twist. Place one hand on the ground or block in between the feet, the other arm up in the air. Twist toward the upper arm side. Repeat on the opposite side.

Ustrasana **(camel)**. Opens the whole front of the body.

Sarvangasana **(shoulderstand).** Blood circulation is increased around the neck and chest, providing treatment for bronchitis, asthma, breathlessness and throat ailments.

Recommended practice after relaxation: *Anuloma Krama* — **segmented inhalation. To practice:**

    1) Exhale deeply, fully.

    2) Inhale the first third of breath in 2-4 seconds, expanding from pubic bone to navel center. Pause.

    3) Inhale second third of breath in 2-4 seconds, expanding from navel center to heart center. Pause.

    4) Inhale last third of breath in 2-4 seconds, expanding from sternum to throat center. Pause.

    5) Exhale slowly and fully.

Repeat for 5 more breaths.

Note: As you inhale, visualize your torso as a tall glass, each breath filling the glass with a bit more water until it's filled to the top. Exhale and pour all the water out.

Practice off the Mat

In any given situation, you have a choice. You have a choice to become the ego self-identity or an enlightened being. You have the choice to be uptight and hardened or relaxed and adaptable.

Wise Words

Keep the brain receptive and observant.

Tune the ears into the vibrations of the exhalation and inhalation.

If we're breathing incorrectly, we're inhibiting our potential for good health.

Visualize taking universal pranic energy in with inhale and releasing toxins on exhale.

All the actions that take place in yoga practice help the breath connect the brain to the heart and, consequently, the world outside to the world within.

Notes

Asanas

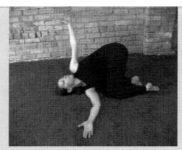

Thread the Needle

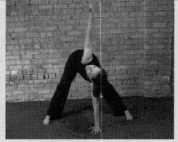

Forward Bend
with Twist

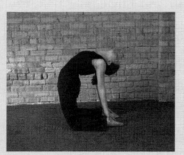

Ustrasana
camel

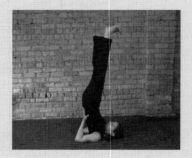

Sarvangasana
shoulderstand

Benefits of *Pranayama*

Intention: To discuss the physical, mental and spiritual attributes of *Pranayama* practice.
Approximate Length: 2 minutes
Pranyama Practice After Relaxation: 5 minutes

Pranayama is the current that removes impurities from our bodies, minds, intellect and ego. The practice of *pranayama* increases our lung capacity so every system in our body benefits. During normal inhalation, an average person takes in about 500 cubic centimeters of air. During deep inhalation, we take in about 6 times as much.

The practice of *pranayama* has countless benefits:

• It purifies the *nadis*, protects the internal organs and cells, and neutralizes lactic acid, which can cause fatigue.

• It relaxes the respiratory muscles of the neck.

• It relaxes the facial muscles. When the face is relaxed, the muscles release their grip over the eyes, ears, nose, tongue and skin — the organs of perception, lessening the tension in the brain. Concentration, calmness and confidence are then present and in control.

• Because the breath is linked to mental and emotional energy, the practice of *pranayama* helps change a negative mental attitude.

• *Pranayama* increases digestion, vitality, perception and memory.

After relaxation, we'll have a *pranayama* practice that includes *nadi shodhana* and *kapalabhati* — the shining skull breath.

Asanas for Deepening

Chest Beating. Make loose fists with the hands and "beat" the upper chest, shoulders, rib cage and side ribs.

Cat Stretch. Feel the movement of breath through spine.
Parshvakonasana **(triangle II).** Stretch from finger tips to toes.
Dangling *Uttanasana* **(standing forward bend).** Feeling the torso swell with inhale and lift slightly, then release on exhale.
Bhujangasana/Shalabhasana/Dhanurasana **(cobra/locust/bow series).** Backbend series to open the breathing passages.

Recommended *pranayama* practice after relaxation:

1 round of *nadi shodhana* **(see p. 62)**
11-22 *kapalabhati* **(shining skull)** breaths. Quick, forceful exhalation with regular inhalations.
1 round of *nadi shodhana* **(begin on passive side)**

Practice off the Mat

If you're feeling tired or dull, a longer inhalation can be a quick pick-me-up; if you need to calm down, a longer exhalation will relax you.

Wise Words

Pranayama: one of the surest ways to attain mastery over the modifications of the mind, making it one-pointed and turning it inward.

With every breath, experience the newness of the now.

Being a yogi is about having the wisdom to remove anything that stifles your consciousness and restricts you to the suffering experience.

Invite your mind to breathe into every part of the body.

Asanas

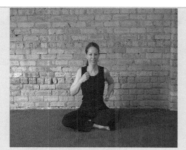

Chest Beating

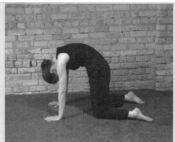
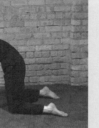

Cat Stretch

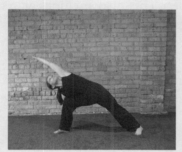

Parshvakonasana
triangle II

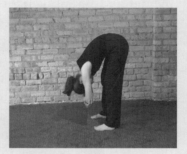

Dangling *Uttanasana*
dangling forward bend

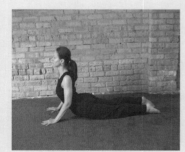

Bhujangasana
cobra

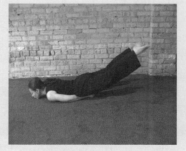

Shalabhasana
locust

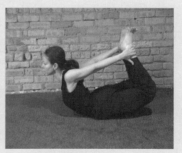

Dhanurasana
bow

Working With *Ha* and *Tha*

Intention: To learn how to balance the lunar and solar manifestations of the body and mind.

Approximate Length: 5 minutes

The essential qualities of *Hatha* Yoga is working with and balancing *ha* and *tha*, the solar and lunar currents representing the dual nature of man: the sun and the moon, male and female, hot and cold, light and dark, mental and physical, right and left. This also includes working with the two major *nadis* that manage our experience of the world. The current that ends in the right nostril, *ida*, and the current that ends in the left nostril, *pingala*.

When we become aware of nostril dominance as we do in the practice of *nadi shodhana*, most of the time one nostril is flowing more freely than the other. But when both nostrils are open, the central current, *sushumna,* is active. This is the most important *nadi* in the body.

The *sushumna* channel or conduit is the pathway to enlightenment, through which awakened energy rises all the way from the core to the crown *chakra*, creating a state of balanced energy. This open pathway has been called "the way to liberation."

Pranayama exercises increase the capacity of the *pranic* body and mind so we can handle the duel nature of the world. We can then more easily move to equilibrium and our naturally peaceful spirit. This is the essence of balancing *ha* and *tha*.

Today, we'll begin practice by working with *ida* and *pingala*. Get into a comfortable sitting position, head, neck and trunk in alignment.

Soften the belly and feel it naturally move with the breath. Now bring your attention to the sensation of breath in the active nostril. Focus on the breath as if it's flowing only through the active side. If thoughts come into your mind, let them go.

Now move your attention to the passive nostril. Feel the touch of breath and focus there without letting the mind wander. Stay here a bit longer than the active side and see if your focused intention opens the passive side.

Finally direct your breath into both nostrils. Inhale from the nostrils inward to the crown. Exhale from the crown to the nostrils. Let your mind relax as you breathe back and forth between these two points.

Asanas for Deepening
Multiply the benefits of your practice by using your full attention.

Squat. Practice 11 breaths of *bhastrika* (bellows breath). You'll notice that a subtle shift in energy can be felt in the nostrils when the *pranic* field is clear.

Padmasana (lotus or 1/2 lotus). *Practice this exercise after 2-3 rounds of* **nadi shodhana** *and the preceding exercise. This is a powerful technique that rapidly alternates the flow of the breath from right to left.*

1) Fold the forearms into the belly.
2) Exhale and fold forward over your arms, bringing the face towards the floor.
3) Inhale deeply and retain the breath as long as comfortable, keeping the spine long, returning to an upright position.
4) Tuck in the chin, close the active nostril, and exhale forcefully through the passive nostril.
5) Inhale through both nostrils and exhale forcefully through the active side. Repeat this exercise until both sides are flowing freely.

Caution: These techniques should not be practiced by anyone with high blood pressure, or chronic problems in the eyes, nasal passages or ears. If you feel dizzy or lightheaded, please stop.

Notes

Notes

Practice off the Mat

Sustaining a balanced *ha* and *tha* can be a helpful approach to your day. For instance, if you need to do quiet work on the computer and feel over-activity in the right nostril, try opening the left. Bring your awareness to the left or try a few rounds of *nadi shodhana* with emphasis on the left channel to activate the right brain. Alternately, if you need to meet with clients, make a presentation, have a social engagement or need external left-brained energy, activate the right nostril.

Wise Words

The place between *ha* and *tha* is where change happens. This is the place of balance and harmony.

Tension restricts the flow of lifeforce. Positive results from *asana* practice can only come from the absence of tension.

When you've reached your edge, don't go beyond it. Instead, pause and breathe there so you can feel the hot and the cold, the good and the bad, the sharp and the soft — attempt to find the mid-ground between *ha* and *tha*.

Asanas

Squat

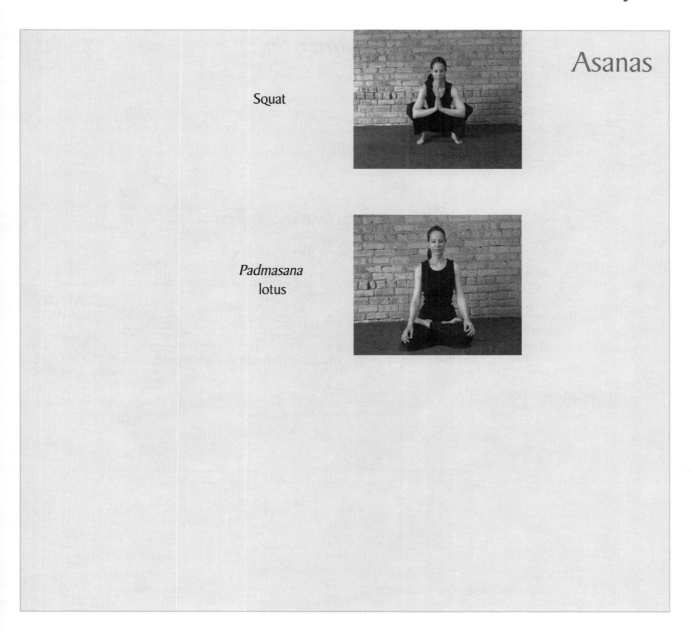

Padmasana
lotus

Chapter Six

On life's journey faith is nourishment,
virtuous deeds are a shelter,
wisdom is the light by day
and right mindfulness is the protection by night.
If a man lives a pure life, nothing can destroy him.

Buddha

Teaching the *Yamas* and *Niyamas*

So much more than a physical discipline, Yoga is a path to liberation rich in ancient philosophy that is as relevant today as it was thousands of years ago. As codified by the Hindu sage, Patanjali, the first two of *Raja* Yoga's eight-limbed path, the *Yamas* and *Niyamas* are ten common-sense guidelines for leading a healthier, happier life. The lessons in this chapter will help explain these sacred values as they relate to work, play, social interaction and the yoga we take to the mat.

Yamas
Moral Disciplines and Restraints

Ahimsa: Non-harming

Be gentle to yourself and all creation. This includes refraining from not only physical violence, but also from criticism and judgment.

Satya: Truthfulness

Avoidance of all falsehood and fabrications.

Asteya: Non-stealing

Do not take or covet what belongs to someone else, whether it be credit for someone's idea or physical objects.

Brahmacharya: Moderation

Avoid excesses in all areas.

Aparigraha: Non-possessiveness

Abstain from greediness, hoarding or possessing beyond one's needs.

Niyamas
Observances

Saucha: Purity
The practice of keeping our minds, hearts and bodies pure.

Santosha: Contentment
Acceptance of life; being satisfied with "what is."

Tapas: Determined Effort
Literally, "that which generates heat." The discipline or "fire" to bring about any kind of change.

Svadhyaya: Self-Study
Study of Self, of scriptures and of the internal states of consciousness.

Ishvara pranidhana: Surrender to the Divine
Living with an awareness of the divine presence. The surrender of ego-driven activities to divine energy.

Yama One
Ahimsa — Non-Violence

Intention: To teach non-violence of self and others. To introduce the first of the five restraints.
Approximate Length: 2 minutes

The five *Yamas*, the first step on the eight-limbed path of *Raja* Yoga, are considered restraints for cultivating happiness and self-confidence to create a better inner and outer world. The first of these is *ahimsa*.

Ahimsa refers to the practice of non-violence. The yogis say there is no higher virtue than non-harming.

Violence isn't limited to killing or hurting another person or animal. It can take many other forms like selfishness, anger or negative words. The place to begin the observance of *ahimsa,* is on ourselves. To paraphrase an ancient Taoist proverb, "If there is to be peace in the world, there must be peace between neighbors. If there is to be peace between neighbors, there must be peace in your heart."

Self-awareness is an important step to see how violence plays out in our existence, from the most subtle, such as self-criticism, to the most obvious manifestations, like war.

Today's practice will focus on *ahimsa* in action and includes the application of patience, compassion and love. Let's set our intention to invite peace and stillness into our individual actions of body and spirit and make a commitment to practice *asana* with *ahimsa*.

Asanas for Deepening

Be kind to yourself. Listen to your edges. Weigh working with effort and working toward pain. Smile. Take pleasure in the posture. Enjoy what

the message of the posture means to your practice of non-violence.
Standing *Yoga Mudra*. Let the weight of the arms open the back muscles. Feel the ribs sliding off your pelvis. Feel the hamstrings and shoulders opening. Release the weight of the world.
Resting *Kapotasana* (pigeon). Never force the openings. Rejecting the beliefs of non-violence and truth to "do" a pose takes you nowhere.

Practice off the Mat

Notice the times in your day when you bring harm to yourself. This could be in the form of self-criticism, angry words, even eating too much or the wrong foods. Then, forgive yourself and rest in the awareness of knowing that the principles of *ahimsa* can be your guiding light of self-love.

Wise Words

Ahimsa comes from awareness of action and thought, the same insight we practice in *asana*.

Ahimsa can be most challenging when applying it to ourselves.

Careful and restrained use of force is sometimes necessary to prevent even greater violence. It is said that in one of his past lives, Buddha killed a man who was about to murder 500 others.

Asana practice is a powerful tool for liberating harmful emotions locked in the body's tissues.

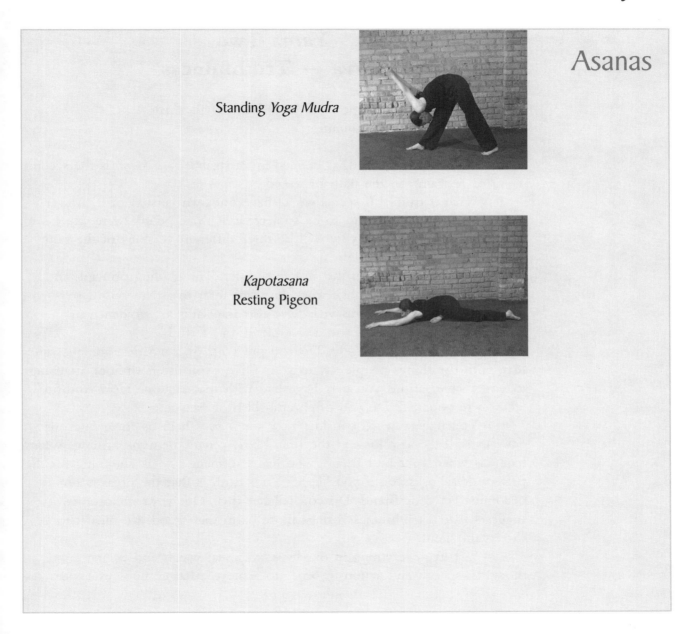

Asanas

Standing *Yoga Mudra*

Kapotasana
Resting Pigeon

Yama Two
Satya — Truthfulness

Intention: To explain yogic truth as defined by Patanjali.
Approximate Length: 4 minutes

Satya or truthfulness, as defined in Patanjali's *Yoga Sutras* is the second *Yama* or restraint on the path of Yoga.

What *is* truth? It seems we all have our own version of it. And although truth is not meant to be subjective, if three people were witness to a car accident, there may very well be three different versions of the same accident.

Truth is more than just not telling lies. The guiding principle in adhering to *satya* is to remove what the yogis refer to as the veil of self-deception. By removing this veil, *satya* also translates as avoidance of distortion, embellishment and any fabrication of truth.

Look at your own life. Do you put your own worries, anxieties and fears into the things people say to you? Or do you listen without attaching to past conversations you may have had with that person? How truthful are you to yourself? Do you often embellish or exaggerate?

You may want to consider how the *Yama*s help us formulate our daily lives. Take at a look at the first *Yama*, *ahimsa*, or non-harming. What happens when your best friend, who has just spent a week shopping for the perfect dress, asks you if you like it? Your truth is that the dress is not becoming on your friend. Do you tell her this? Our yoga philosophy suggests that if truthfulness brings more harm than good, we must choose to remain silent.

Just like everything in our lives, we must weigh and balance thoughts, speech and action in order to achieve a harmonious existence.

Today, notice the truth in your practice. Do you tell yourself you can't do a pose even if you've never tried it? Do you tell yourself a posture doesn't cause pain when it does?

Practice *satya* — working with honesty. The liberating effects of *asana* require careful inner listening. Truthfulness is a remarkable tool for purifying our energies.

Asana for Deepening

Keep honesty present in your practice. Ask yourself the meaningful questions. Is it true your mind is wandering? Is it true you feel anxiety in a pose? Notice how *prana* is enhanced or cut off by a change in mental attitude.

Vrikshasana (tree). Relax into the holding of balance as you observe the responses between your outer body and your will and ego.

Virasana (hero). Be alert to the truth of your skeletal system, including your ankles, feet, knees, thighs and sitbones. Feel your weight sink toward the floor.

Pashchimottanasana (posterior stretch). Notice any demand in your mind that suggests you should be where you're not organically ready to be. Enjoy the honesty and integrity of this complete "stretch of the west."

Practice off the Mat

Sharpen your listening skills. Can other people's words take us from our own truth?

When my kids were quite young, an older friend told me to cherish every moment with my children, they soon will grow and move on to their own families. Was she suggesting I was asleep at the maternal wheel? That I did

Notes

131

Notes

not appreciate my children? Or was I simply diluting her words with my own defenses? When I listened with *satya*, I really heard what she was saying, which was simply to enjoy this time in my life. True listening is our ability to surrender to another's words.

How often have you projected your own "truths" into someone else's words?

Wise Words

When body and mind are in sync, truth rises to the top.

Take time to listen for inner truth.

Telling the truth has little meaning until we first remove the veil of illusion.

In yoga, as awareness expands, our perception becomes clearer, and we come closer to the truth, seeing life as it is in each moment.

Asanas

Vrikshasana
tree

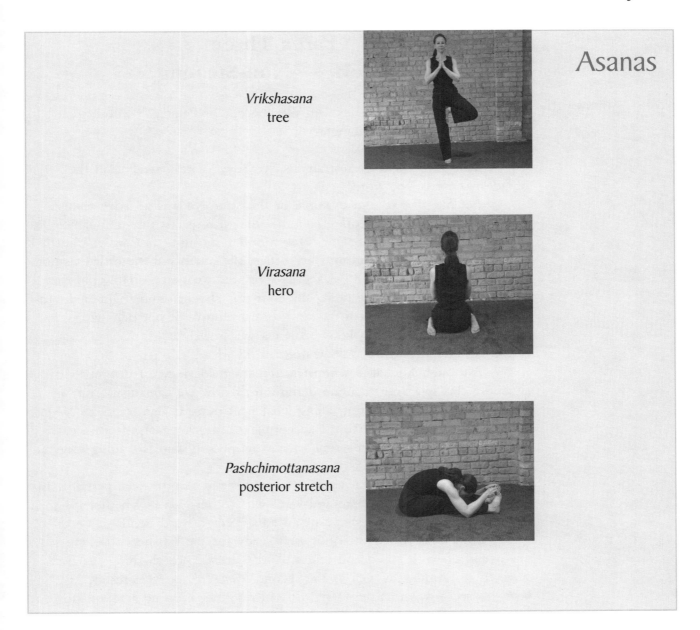

Virasana
hero

Pashchimottanasana
posterior stretch

Yama Three
Asteya — Non-Stealing

Intention: To define and explain the concept of Patanjali's *asteya.*
Approximate Length: 2 minutes

The third *Yama* or restraint is the *Yama* of non-stealing in the broadest sense of the word.

Let me give you an example of this. Carolyn was an advertising agency copywriter who worked side-by-side with an art director named Michael to create ad campaigns. One Monday morning as Carolyn shuffled passed the agency staff and into her office, she overheard the office clamor. "We were robbed over the weekend! What did they take? How did they break in?" Abuzz with the news, the staff was shocked and frightened. Just as Carolyn sat at her desk to take a quick inventory of her belongings, her partner, Michael, who was known for his wit as well as his designs, came screaming into her office, "They stole all my ideas!"

Although Michael's whimsical remark made light of the tense situation, this is a very accurate definition of how we can misuse *asteya.* *Asteya* doesn't just mean not taking what isn't ours. It also refers to *taking credit* for things that aren't ours, accepting too much change from a cashier, being late and thus "stealing time" from the person who is waiting for you, and, yes, even stealing ideas.

Think about all the ways *asteya* may relate to our *asana* practice. In yoga class, we often compare and want what others have. Whether it's their flexibility, strength, body shape or an advanced forward bend.

Sometimes when the body isn't ready for the finished pose, we might end up with strain and injury. And there we are violating the first *Yama,* non-harming, as well as the second *Yama,* truth. As a result, we begin to see how the *Yamas* build on one another, creating a foundation for life.

Asanas for Deepening

Practice postures that are challenging, if not impossible for you. Treasure the fact that you can bend forward, although you may need to bend your knees.

Let go of the craving to do a pose like someone else. Pick a headstand, the splits, crow or balance postures that are out of reach today. Make each posture your own and appreciate what you can do.

Practice off the Mat

Think about all the ways you may steal and not recognize it. Do you use office supplies for personal use? Do you use more natural resources than you need? Do you steal from nature?

Appreciate all the things you have. When we look outside ourselves for more, we neglect the riches of our lives. Foster a sense of abundance in your life.

Wise Words

Don't steal energy from others. Just think of someone who always "drains" you when they're around.

Cultivate a sense of completeness and self-sufficiency. Let go of cravings.

Notes

Yama Four
Brahmacharya — Moderation

Intention: To introduce moderation in all aspects of living.
Approximate Length: 3 minutes

Imagine reaching for your third candy bar and the voice in your head says, "Everything in moderation." That's the foundation of *bramacharya* — moderation, the fourth of the *Yamas*.

Brahmacharya is commonly translated as celibacy. But its real meaning. Its real meaning is to stop the wasting of one's energies.

Patanjali's *Yoga Sutras* say, when one is established in *brahmacharya* or non-indulgence, one is endowed with inexhaustible energy.

Think about the things you indulge in: food, drink, caffeine, sleep, work, play, exercise, feeling depressed — it goes on and on. As the saying goes, " Too much of anything is no longer good."

As yogis, we practice moment-to-moment awareness and inner clarity to expand on the bigger awareness of life. It's this very process that allows us to respond to our true needs, as we carefully listen to divine guidance and follow the path of moderation.

Brahmacharya on the yoga mat often teaches a new perspective to our poses. We begin to explore the hows and whys of poses we indulge in and those we resist. Many of us spend most of our practice in poses that come easy and resist the ones that are challenging.

In today's practice, try each pose as though you've never attempted it before with a fresh, open mind and receptive body. Use a beginner's mind: there is no past, no future, only what is happening right now.

Listen and trust the voice within that always seeks balance, harmony and peace in every movement and moment. As you let go of the bonds of the pleasures and pains of the past, you just might discover hidden abilities, new energies and playfulness in your practice.

Asanas for Deepening

Practice any variation of **Surya Namaskara (sun salutation)** with respect for divine light above and within. Ask your inner spark what would feel just right? Where is the *brahmacharya* within my *Surya Namaskara*? *Brahmacharya* is dedication to the perception, understanding and awareness of divinity.

Practice moderation without spending too much energy on any one pose. Coordinate holding postures with the process of moving through them with breath. Make sure to include poses that you normally resist, such as **Chaturanga (stick)** or **3-Legged Adho Mukha Shvanasana (3–legged downdog).**

Practice off the Mat

Practice *brahmacharya* by meeting each moment fresh and new. Experience the power and magic in the moment while going to work, hugging a loved one or taking a deep breath.

Before taking that third piece of candy or drink, sleeping too long or too little, or surrounding yourself with toxic people, remember: "Everything in moderation."

Most yoga masters argue against casual sex. You don't have to switch off your sexuality, just make each sexual experience count. Involve awareness of the heart. Sexual satisfaction begins with an open heart and blossoms through awareness.

Notes

Notes

Wise Words

Do you eat in moderation, think in moderation, talk in moderation and do all activities in moderation?

Work toward awareness of both energy and balance to avoid an emotional seesaw which can create overindulgence.

When our inner and outer lives are balanced, the mind becomes calm, our natural serenity flows and we feel content with life.

Asanas

Surya Namaskara
sun salutation
(see p.101 for basic 12 poses)

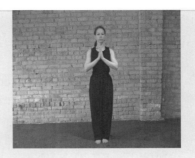

Chaturanga
stick

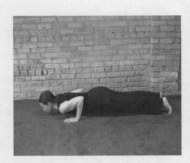

Adho Mukha Shvanasana
3-legged downdog

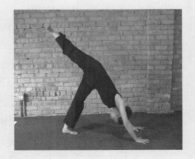

Yama Five
Aparigraha — Non-Possessiveness

Intention: To learn to recognize greed within ourselves.
Approximate Length: 2 minutes

Aparigraha or non-possessiveness, is the fifth of the *Yamas* or yogic restraints. From a yogic point of view, possessiveness or greed is a vacant search for happiness, because whatever possessions you acquire will never fulfill you.

Buying, wanting or accepting more than is necessary clouds the mind and keeps it from understanding the deeper motivations and reasons for life.

So what *is* really necessary and appropriate for us to be healthy, happy and fulfilled? Ask yourself: do you really need all the clothes, toys or trinkets in your house? How much of it has become clutter?

The more possessions we have and the more attached we become to our things, the more our environments and minds become muddled and busy. You can see how easy it is to lose your perspective and connection to what life is truly about.

Moreover, it's important to open your mind to the possibility that you may be attached to people such as your children, your spouse or your friends. When this happens, there's no space to step back and simply appreciate the essence in that being.

Likewise, we can be possessive with our thoughts. We hold onto our own ideas, our principles, our way of doing things. Some consider this a state of inflexibility that can transfer to our muscles and tissues.

The secret to *aparigraha* is learning to let go. Letting go of attachment to possessions, people, thoughts or a set way of doing things.

Aparigraha often shows up in *asana* practice. Some people are attached to doing a perfect pose or doing a pose a certain way. Others may

Notes

be attached to old tensions or injuries, or to a particular spot in the classroom.

Our challenge today is to detach from the posture, the outcome, the way you think you are. Let go of your attachment to the practice or the way you want it to be. This way, you can let the possibilities flourish.

Asanas for Deepening

When we attach to our strains and injuries, we block the natural flow of circulation in the muscles. When encountering tightness, use breath awareness to create balance and space.

Let go of expectations of how our bodies should perform, or how a pose should be practiced or taught.

Only by letting go of ideas can we be open and receptive to the deeper experience of yoga. Each time we undertake *asana* is a brand new beginning.

Shavasana (corpse). Begin and end your practice with shavasana. Practice with total detachment. Lie down and let go of outer tensions, muscles and limbs. Let go of senses and thoughts so you can be who you really are.

Rag Doll. This stretch for the hamstrings and back teaches us about the power of letting go. Hang effortlessly and tune into the vibrations originating in the spine. Feel it spread throughout the torso. This variation of *Uttanasana* is one of the ultimate surrender poses because *it* works *you*, not the other way around.

Gomukhasana (cow's face). Surrender your weight to the ground. Add the arms, but don't attach to getting the "attachment" of your fingers behind the back.

Notes

Practice off the Mat

Do you have too much "stuff"? Are you overly attached to your partner or child? Are you envious of your neighbors? What happens when you *don't* get what you want? Loosen your grasp on material possessions and let go of the ego, which is doing the gripping.

When we let go of something, someone, or some expectation, we create space in our lives for new energies to come in. Only when we permit ourselves to let go of some idea of how life *has* to be, can the moment truthfully transpire.

Wise Words

The man who knows when enough is enough will always have enough.

The yoga practitioner who is well-trained in the art of greedlessness is said to understand the deeper reasons for life.

Don't cling to a person, place or thing thinking that's going to bring you happiness.

Asanas

Shavasana
corpse

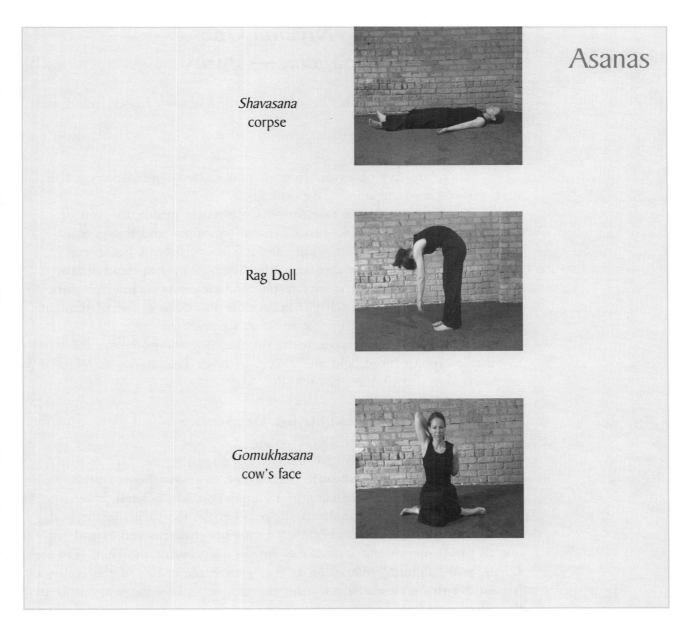

Rag Doll

Gomukhasana
cow's face

Niyama One
Saucha — Purity

Intention: To introduce the *Niyamas*; to define *saucha* of body, mind and spirit.
Approximate Length: 1-2 minutes

There are five observances or *Niyamas* in yoga philosophy. The first one is *saucha,* meaning self-purification.

Saucha is not only a foundation for physical health; the aim of *saucha* is to cleanse the mind of its negative emotions and thoughts.

As the mind works toward calmness and clarity, it becomes conscious of any toxins or disease in the body. Body and mind always work hand in hand. That is why fasting and cleansing techniques alone won't necessarily produce self-purification. If the mind is full of thoughts, concerns and "mental garbage," it must also come clean.

We'll focus our practice today on cleansing the body and the mind to make room for more light and energy to flow. This allows us to focus on awakening our divine light within.

Asanas for Deepening

Squat. Stimulates the digestive track.
***Sarvangasana* (shoulderstand)**. The change in gravity helps lymph drainage and stimulates digestion and elimination. In general, inversions by the nature of being "upside down" help loosen all the toxins in the body.
***Simhasana* (lion)**. 1) Sit on heels. 2) Come up on knees and extend arms out. 3) Open mouth and stretch the tongue out towards the chin. On the exhale, roar "ahhhhh" like a lion as you gaze at the center of the eyebrows. Repeat 2-3 times. *Simhasana* cleanses the tongue and removes toxins from the throat and breath.

Parivrtta Trikonasana (revolved triangle)/*Marichyasana* (seated twist). The squeeze and soak action of twisting postures cleanses the organs. The "squeezing" forces out toxins and waste while the "soaking" releases fresh blood, bathing the cells with oxygen and nutrients.

Practice off the Mat

For the mind to be clear, the body, as well as the surroundings of the body, (home, office, practice space, yoga mat) must be clean.

In general, keep your home and work area clean. Don't let dirty dishes, laundry, unread mail or garbage pile up.

Bathe once a day and, if possible, move your bowels once a day. If the system is sluggish, toxins stay trapped in your body, keeping tension, anger, and slothfulness locked within the tissues. If your system is slow, practice deeper, longer held twists such as supine twists before getting out of bed, drink eight glasses of water a day, avoid white flours and load up on fibrous foods.

Wise Words

The body, breath and mind have an automatic cleansing process. The breath ebbs and flows, thoughts enter and leave constantly. On every level, waste is being released and replaced with energy and light.

From a yogic perspective, the accumulations of internal wastes is the primary cause of disease.

Notes

Asanas

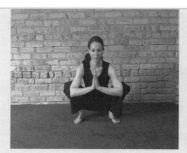
Squat

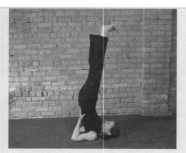
Sarvangasana
shoulderstand

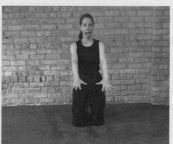
Simhasana
lion

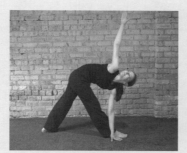
Parivrtta Trikonasana
revolved triangle

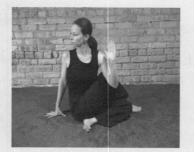
Marichyasana
seated twist

Niyama Two
Santosha — Contentment

Notes

Intention: To teach the significance of acceptance and choice as it relates to contentment of daily living.
Approximate Length: 3 minutes

Santosha or contentment, is the second *Niyama* or observance in yogic philosophy. We tend to think of contentment as the fulfillment of desires, but the yogis tell us that this kind of happiness is short-lived. And, as we learn from the *Yama aparigraha* — non-possessiveness, desires create more desires and more cravings. Like a well that can never be filled, greed is a vacant search for happiness.

The yogi's view of contentment develops from an experience of acceptance of whatever life has brought to us. Contentment is mindfulness of living in the moment, something we naturally apply in *asana*.

There's a parable about two women who, from an outsider's perspective, seemed to live quite similar lives. Both were the same age, had the same-sized home, same-sized family, and same income level. The two women even looked somewhat alike. There was only one real difference: one woman was quite satisfied with her life, while the other felt empty and frustrated. As we see from this parable, happiness, the feeling of contentment, is a choice.

Once you decide that whatever you have in this moment is all you need, contentment will *always* find a place in your life.

Santosha requires a sense of inner acceptance which begins when you stop comparing yourself with others. As long as there's comparison accompanied by judgment, there cannot be contentment.

Today in our *asana* practice, let's accept what we have. Let's accept what brought us here today. And let's accept our bodies, abilities and limitations as they are right now. And enjoy the journey!

Asanas for Deepening

Personal practice will help you accept your body as it is and allow you to lose your classroom competitive edge.

***Trikonasana* (triangle).** Witness the breath flowing into the awkward spaces. Stay in the pose and watch your body unfold through breath, time and patience.   If something feels disagreeable, stay unattached to outcome and observe whether what you feel is pain, curious sensation, or emotional discomfort. Does *santosha* arise, even for a moment?

***Setu Bandha Sarvangasana* (bridge).** Bridge allows us to open our hearts and thus our experience to the truth and beauty of our inner and outer worlds. The posture keeps us from shutting out the reality of our actual needs and enjoying the sensation of the present. Let yourself be freed from the past so you can experience the gratification of the now.

***Natarajasana* (king dancer).** Feel the cause and effect, the ebb and flow, the strength and flexibility of the pose. Notice how *prana* moves you, creating more space in your field of energy. Conversely, does the breath struggle, thereby blocking energy flow and shutting you down? The choice is yours. Don't hassle yourself if you're not as balanced or aligned as you think you should be. Where are you resisting? Where is there movement? Where is there a feeling of peace?

Depression Flow. A quick fix for the everyday blues. Practice moving from ***Urdhva Mukha Shvanasana* (updog)** to ***Adho Mukha Shvanasana* (downdog)** on the breath (inhale into updog, exhale to downdog) 6 to 20 times.

Practice off the Mat

The purpose of contentment is to help us see that we're exactly where we're supposed to be right now. Know that there is something to learn from everything, everyone, and every experience that crosses your path.

Notes

Make sure you find the time to experience the things that give you a happy feeling. Ask yourself how contentment shows up in your life. Is it taking a walk in the woods? Is it resting in the sun? Is it enjoying a cup of coffee with a friend? Is it holding hands with someone you love?

Practice *santosha* by remembering the blessings you have in your life each day. There are thousands of things all around you that are extraordinary if you choose to look at them that way.

Wise Words

Happiness is a way of travel, not a destination.

Contentment brings us into the very moment, bringing a sense of happiness into our lives right now.

Santosha means to free the mind of the mundane — the trivial irritations of life that take up too much of our spirit. When we can let go of our daily technicalities, we see life in a larger context with detachment and inner balance.

Accept what you have and enjoy what you have. Only by acceptance can we ever find contentment.

Contentment allows us to know that whatever we are doing, we're making the right choice for ourselves.

Asanas

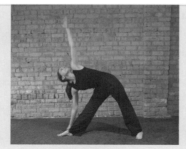

Trikonasana
triangle

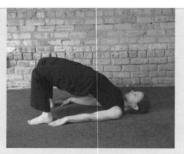

Setu Bandha Sarvangasana
bridge

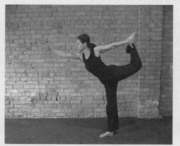

Natarajasana
king dancer

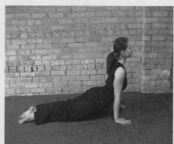

Urdhva Mukha Shvanasana
updog

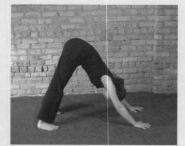

Adho Mukha Shvanasana
downdog

Niyama Three
Tapas — Passionate Commitment and Discipline

Intention: To define *tapas*; to employ whatever it takes to attain a necessary goal.
Approximate Length: 2 minutes

Tapas, the third of the *Niyamas* or observances in yoga philosophy, is defined as the willingness to do whatever is necessary to reach a goal.

Tapas is about austerity, sacrifice and discipline. Its meaning is "heat" or "fire" and therefore *tapas* refers to the fire that brings forth transformation. When we describe someone working very hard at something, we refer to that as having "the fire" in the belly.

According to the sages, the fire that's created through yoga practice destroys pollution in one's consciousness and leads to the control of the body and senses. Therefore, there can be no yoga without *tapas*.

Consequently, to create change on any level — whether it's to lose weight, change jobs, achieve *hanumanasana* (splits) or attain enlightenment, requires a constant commitment to *tapas*.

A requirement of *tapas* is to cut through distractions and bring our full attention to the present moment. To apply *tapas*, we might begin by observing the quality of mindfulness that we bring to any given activity. How often do we focus 100 percent of the time?

When we apply *tapas* to our *asana* practice, we can open up to a whole new level of discrimination. We don't practice mechanically doing the same poses with the same intensity every day. Instead we practice mindfully with determined effort to create change.

Asanas for Deepening

Be the pose. Exercise your awareness as you exercise your body. Put the effort in, and you'll get the change you need.

Plank. Visualize a flame at the navel center as you hold the pose. Expand the internal fire with your focus and breath. Notice the feeling of heat, strength and power.

Parsvakonasana **(triangle II — with or without arm wrap).** Keep weight on the balls of feet. Spread the shoulder blades and spine long from the back of the skull. Move energy from the pelvic floor into the navel center. Inhale and bring vitality and lifeforce into the whole body. Exhale and guide that force throughout your body.

Fire Series (leg lifts). Keep the concentration on the navel center while continuing to fuel the fire of *tapas*. There are several variations of the fire series. They can be practiced on the elbows or for more challenging classes, lying on the back with navel center pressed to lumber spine, lumbar spine pressed to the ground. Some examples of this series include single and double leg lifts, bicycle leg movements, leg circles, horizontal and vertical scissors and ***Jathara Parivartanasana*** **(leg lifts with twist).**

Practice off the Mat

Tapas may be summed up as "where there is a will, there is a way." If you often say to yourself, "I want to practice yoga daily and I will find time for it," this will is the *tapas*.

Will yourself to make one small change in your life everyday. For instance, you may want to drink an extra glass of water every afternoon, call your mother, or simply commit to washing your dishes every night.

Find what you need to will in your life and commit yourself to the fire of *tapas*.

Wise Words

Long sitting meditation is a disciplined practice during which physical heat is generated. This physical heat burns the ego away to reveal the true inner spirit.

Tapas is stirred by the internal knowledge that life is a gift and one should make the most of it.

Yoga is about being able to purify and undo anything that may hold you down and restrict you to the suffering experience.

Without self-discipline, one's actions, words and thoughts become scattered and *prana* becomes weakened.

Notes

Asanas

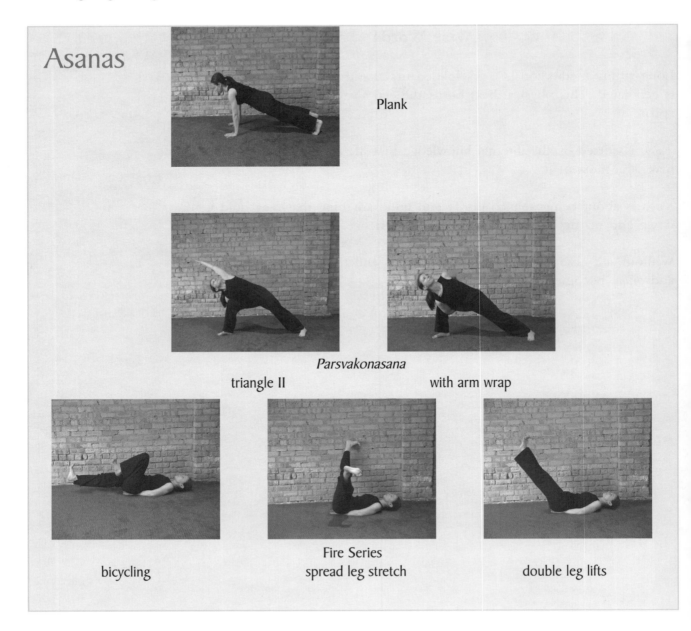

Plank

Parsvakonasana

triangle II   with arm wrap

bicycling

Fire Series
spread leg stretch   double leg lifts

Niyama Four
Svadhyaya — Self-Study

Intention: To define *svadhyaya*: to search out the meaning of spiritual concepts through self-study, questioning, and experience in relation to all of life.
Approximate Length: 2 minutes

Today we're going to discuss the fourth *Niyama* or observance — *svadhyaya*, which means self-study or self-observation. The practice of self-study refers to both the understanding of the Self through the study of sacred texts as well as the skill of self-observation that leads to yoga or unification.

Svadhyaya is the effort to know the Self, the inner self as well as the outer Self of universal consciousness.

One method of self-study is with writings that inspire us to feel the presence of the inner spirit. We can then apply these inspirations to our lives so it has meaning to us.

In our *asana* practice, *svadhyaya* helps us observe moment to moment changes in our body and mind. How are you feeling in your body? Is your mind present? What subject matter draws your mind away? Applying *svadhyaya* to the yoga postures is one way of looking within and connecting to your inner truth.

Today, as we practice and move and focus, go inside. Pause between your postures, listen and learn from them. They have much to teach you. Be honest about what it is you don't know or don't quite understand and let yourself learn through the experience.

Asanas for Deepening

Practice self-study through breath awareness. Turn your attention inward and become aware of your breathing. Imagine and feel how the breath allows spaces in all the abstract places in every part of the body to open and vibrate within. Feel the *prana,* the lifeforce, activating every layer of consciousness.

***Gomukhasana* (cow's face).** Almost everyone has a definitive response to this pose. Do your fingertips reach each other? Are your hips opening for the first time? How can gravity help you release further?

***Bhujangasana* (cobra).** Observe how *prana* runs up the front of the spine and down the legs. Notice the chest opening, breath moving into the upper lungs. Relax in ***Makarasana* (crocodile)** and feel the back tingle and the shift in energy and mood.

***Upavistha Konasana* (seated angle).** Use this posture to gently expand your self-knowledge. Take yourself to your limit through astute awareness and physical and mental adjustments. Study the pose without stepping back from or going over the edge. Challenge yourself to stay mindful.

Practice off the Mat

Remind yourself to practice constant self-observation and self-study in daily living. Every movement is an *asana*, every breath is *pranayama*, every thought meditation.

Before retiring each night ask yourself, "what did I learn today?"

Wise Words

Svadhyaya gives you pause to breathe, relax, feel, and learn. Be open to receive and enjoy the spirit of exploration within you.

Study and practice go hand in hand. Acquire some useful yoga reference books and scriptures such as Patanjali's *Yoga Sutras*, *Hatha* Yoga *Pradipika*, and the *Bhagavad Gita*. As you study, discover how the concepts in these books change over time as you uncover the deeper meanings of life.

Notes

Asanas

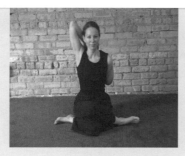

Gomukhasana
cow's face

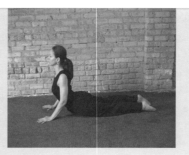

Bhujangasana
cobra

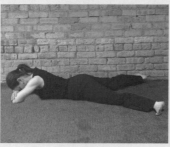

Makarasana
crocodile

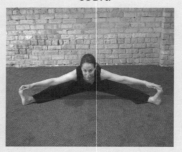

Upavistha Konasana
seated angle

Niyama Five
Ishvara Pranidhana —
Surrender to God/Light/Energy of the Universe

Intention: To practice with faith and dedication to the divine energy of the universe.
Approximate Length: 2 minutes

The fifth *Niyama* or yoga observance is *ishvara pranidhana*. This observance engages your relationship to the divine energy of the universe. *Ishvara pranidhana* is honoring a higher ideal or spiritual consciousness in your life.

When you surrender your ego-driven activities to divine spirit, doorways open for positive energy to flow into all areas of your life. According to the sages, by uniting your individual self with that of a higher principle, be it God, Buddha, Jesus or nature itself, egotism, trivialities and selfishness are removed.

Every action we take can be done with significance, every word we speak with meaning and truth, and every thought with clarity.

Today, take your practice within, find out the truth of who and what you are. Offer the fruits of yourself, your work, and your love to the divine spirit or spark within. Notice what a difference it makes when you surrender your ego and completely free yourself to something bigger than yourself.

Asanas for Deepening

When we practice *asana* with a sense of devotion to a higher purpose, it becomes a vehicle for positive energy to permeate our lives. We relax and become more genuine and receptive in our practice.

***Namaste* Circles.** Sit in **Easy Pose** and move the arms up and over the head and in circles out to the sides with palms connecting in *namaste* over heart. Inhale and move arms outward, exhale as hands move to heart. Feel the universal spirit within the heart center.

Tripod. Top of head on the ground, hands under shoulders, fingers spread. For a more challenging variation, lift knees on to the "shelf" of the forearms. This posture helps to awaken the crown *chakra*, our connection to divine consciousness located at the top of the head.

Standing Squat. Bring the hands in *namaste* over heart. Feel the connectedness in the feet and legs. Bring both earth and heaven energy into the heart center.

Practice off the Mat

Meditate on what you do each day, who you talk to, where your mind goes, how your body moves. Start your meditation from when you wake, brush your teeth, eat your breakfast, go to work and on through the rest of your day. How does *ishvara pranidhana* weave into your daily activities?

Wise Words

The practice of *ishvara pranidhana* is a way of living in which you are always aware of the divinity, of the supreme intelligence.

It is wonderfully illuminating to connect our small lives with the larger whole.

Asanas

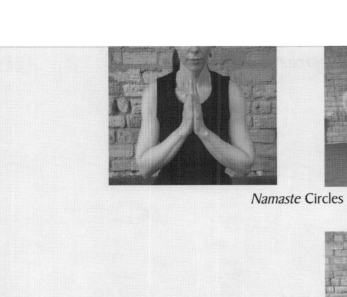 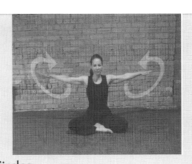

Namaste Circles

Tripod

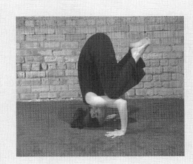

Standing Squat

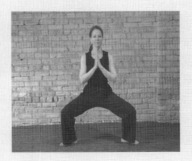

Chapter Seven

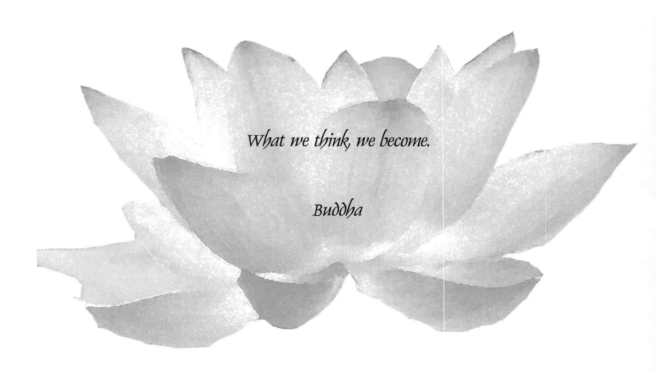

What we think, we become.

Buddha

Emotions

The definition of yoga *asana* is a position that is both steady and comfortable; a place where one can feel completely present. Those who are both present and still learn how agitated the mind states can be. Practice then becomes a purifying method of listening to the inner workings of the mind and emotions.

The lessons that follow will allow you to recognize the emotions that come up during practice so that you can become more aware of them during your day.

Don't criticize yourself if you find that negative emotions seem to lead the way. Just look, listen, and be aware. When we're able to work with the emotional side of yoga *asana*, we become more sensitized, perceptive, and responsive, so that we can make the appropriate changes.

Pay Attention.

Emotional Effects of *Asana*

Intention: To present yoga's harmonizing effects on emotions.
Approximate Length: 2 minutes

Have you ever noticed the effect your yoga practice has had on your emotions? It's like a welcome sense of spaciousness, as though you've just cleaned a room in your mind and swept away the dirt. You've opened up the curtains and let the sun shine on your inner self so that healing, along with light, can come shining through.

Usually, the positive emotions come to the surface: our sense of humor, patience, concentration. As we surrender and let go of frustrations, fear and worry, we start to feel like our "old selves" again.

The flip side of this, of course, is when the *negative* emotions come up and stay with us. Quite naturally, if we're doing what we're supposed to be doing — cleansing and releasing — feeling our negative emotions are paramount to our whole renewing process.

When this happens, give yourself space to feel what you're feeling. Instead of suppressing these emotions, realize that these feelings came up for a purpose. Then do your best to stay mindful of them, giving them enough space so you can eventually free them from your spirit.

Our poses can highly influence our emotional states. For instance, because of the expansive inhalation and opening of the chest, backbending, traditionally a stimulating practice, can equalize a low mood. Exhale-intensive poses like forward bends tend to calm an agitated mind. In any balanced practice, both inhale-oriented and exhaled-oriented postures are executed to create equilibrium in the body and breath and lend us control of our emotional harmony.

Today's focus is on restoring equipoise, empowering us to release emotionally and make positive changes in our layers of consciousness.

Asanas for Deepening

Sarvangasana/Halasana (shoulderstand/plow). Helps reverse energy blocks on many levels — inflexible thinking, stuck emotions, feelings of sadness.

Child's Pose. Sends relaxing signals to both sympathetic and parasympathetic nervous systems.

Garudasana (eagle). Offers relief of the scattered mind. Works on balance of external and internal worlds.

Marichyasana (half spinal twist). One of yoga's greatest harmonizers, as it both calms the mind and releases any sluggishness in the body.

Janu Shirshasana (head-to-knee forward bend pose). Relieves feelings of anxiety, fearfulness and stress. On each exhalation, let the torso sink further toward the legs.

Dhanurasana (bow). Helps stimulate the inhale, arouses adrenal glands.

Woodchopper. Assists in the emotional release of frustration and anger. Stand, lift your imaginary ax on inhale, and with a forceful "HA" on the exhale, chop the imaginary wood between your legs.

Practice off the Mat

Notice the things in your life that cause you to tense up. Are you a tense driver, talker or worker? When you cook or do the dishes, does your back feel strain? Whether it's in the shoulders, neck, back or navel center, practice every day moment-to-moment body awareness. This will help you cleanse your negative emotions and trapped issues so they don't find a permanent home in your body.

Notes

Notes

Wise Words

The path of yoga can cut through the roots of suffering.

Hatha Yoga teaches us control of breath and control of body. Through awareness, we learn concentration, control of our thought patterns and emotional control. The serious yoga practitioner will cling less to life's negative matters, permitting the practice to have a leveling effect on the whole emotional body.

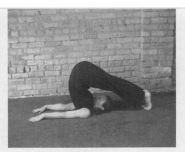

Sarvangasana
shoulderstand

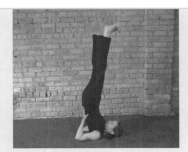

Halasana
plow

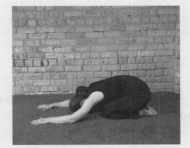

Child's Pose

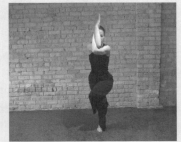

Garudasana
eagle

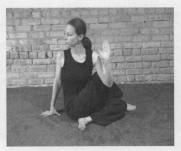

Marichyasana
seated twist

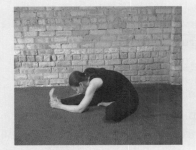

Janu Shirshasana
head-to-knee

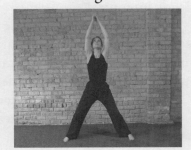

Woodchopper

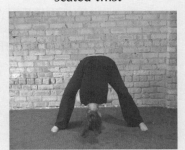

167

Frustration in the Body

Intention: To bring awareness to how the body manifests frustration.
Approximate Length: 2 minutes

When we feel frustrated, this generally means we're not flowing with the experiences of our lives. Instead we're pushing away or resisting something. Frustration then collects in the body. Many of us feel it in the shoulders, the neck, low back, and the hips.

Problems in the shoulders represent irritability and resistance to change.

Issues in the back can be related to some repression or restriction in your life, or the feeling of carrying the weight of the world.

Repressed anger creates tension in the neck as you force your feelings down your throat instead of saying what you want to say. You can literally experience a *pain in the neck* from something or someone who makes you angry.

The hips are related to general frustration. Notice the person who often stands with her hands on her hips. This is a gesture of feeling frustrated and not in control.

Through a balanced *asana* practice and particularly the postures that work on these specific areas, many of our frustrations can be released. Let's set our intentions for today's practice to work out any frustration that has manifested or threatens to manifest itself in any of these areas.

Please lie in *shavasana*. Breathe deeply into your belly, totally putting all of your awareness into the breath. Feel all the emotions of your respiratory system: the air in the nostrils, throat and chest, and the belly and chest rising. Feel the rib cage expanding out to the front, to the sides beneath the armpits and all the way into the lower back. Gently move your attention from your mental state to your breath, so you can observe and step back from your emotions.

Asanas for Deepening

Reclining Knee Twist. Works on releasing frustration in hips. Lie on the back. Stretch arms out to sides shoulder height, palms down. Inhale and bend left knee to chest. Exhale and twist to your right side, releasing a deep sigh (AHHHH). Inhale, return to the back. Practice 3 times on each side. This twist is also beneficial for sciatica, headaches and low back stiffness.
Cat Stretch. Releases frustration in the back, pelvic floor, abdomen, and back of the neck.
Neck Stretches. There are several variations to practice: ear to shoulder, look over the shoulder, drop chin to chest, neck rolls.
Shoulder Work. Can be done seated or standing.

    1) **Arm Circles.** Hold a strap about shoulders' width distance apart. Inhale bring arms forward and up toward the sky; exhale, bring arms behind you, using the full range of motion in the shoulders.

    2) **Arm Pulls.** Raise right arm up, bringing the right arm alongside the right ear. Reach the left arm down and outward, stretching through the fingers. Inhale and energize upward through the right arm and exhale as you reach outward through the left arm and hand. Practice several breaths before changing arms.

    3) **Collarbone Stretch**. Interlace hands behind you, open the chest, and bring the knuckles to the left side of the waist. Feel the right shoulder blade coming in toward the spine. Roll the shoulders back while squeezing elbows together. Change sides.
***Naukasana* (reclining boat)**. Works on the acupressure points related to general body frustration, body aches, digestive problems, and fear. Lie on the abdomen with the chin on floor. Stretch the arms straight out in front of you. Slowly and deeply inhale, lift the arms, chest, head and legs off the ground, arching the back. Hold for 3-6 breaths. Relax in **Child's Pose**.

Notes

Notes

Practice off the Mat

Body language has so much to do with how you express your emotions. Do you hunch your shoulders in an effort to protect or shield yourself? Do you often settle your hands on your hips? Notice your emotional frustration and then recognize how it manifests in your body.

Wise Words

The more we let go and release in all areas of our life, the more life unfolds itself to us.

With daily practice, patience and faith, energy blocks will diminish, inviting health, healing and lifeforce into your being.

Each new breath is a new moment of life. The practice is to find the newness in each moment.

All your issues are in your tissues.

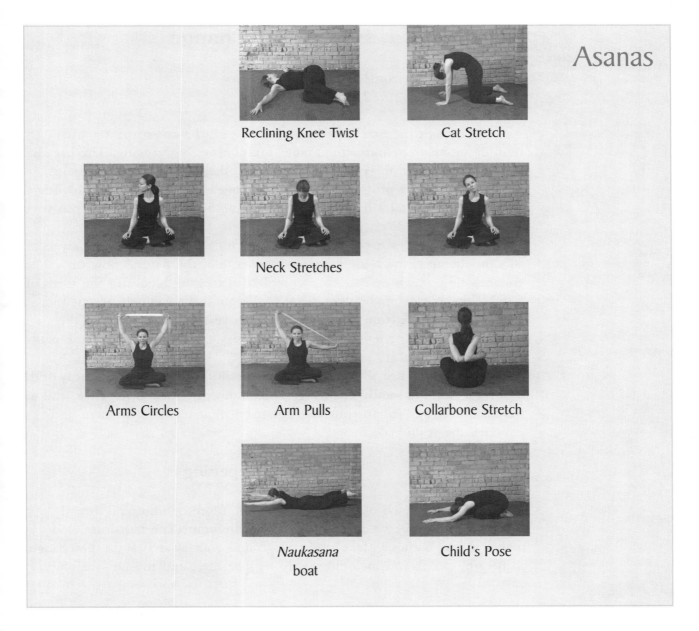

Asanas

Reclining Knee Twist

Cat Stretch

Neck Stretches

Arms Circles

Arm Pulls

Collarbone Stretch

Naukasana
boat

Child's Pose

Embracing Change

Intention: To welcome change into our lives.
Approximate Length: 2 minutes

Through the practice of yoga, we begin to awaken to how life unfolds moment by moment. Things are constantly changing. The breath, your state of mind, the phases of the moon, the changing of the seasons. This can be both a profound revelation — life is like a flower that blooms continuously — and a harsh reminder that nothing lasts forever. Even your body will let you down in the end.

When we resist change, the ego will try to hold on to the body as it is. Consequently, the body contracts, tenses, and the natural flow of energies slow down or may stop completely, creating blocks in the form of a tight hip or frozen shoulder. That's why, until we willingly accept the changes that occur from day to day, year to year, and surrender to the natural course of existence, very little progress can be made along the path of yoga.

Asana practice shows us how our bodies, our minds, and the world around us are constantly changing. Today, through breath, patience, and a watchful eye, we'll honor our changes from movement to moment and embrace the reality of change.

Asanas for Deepening

From the first stretch of the morning to the more mindful and heated **Surya Namaskara**, we can feel and sense the immediate transformation it makes in our bodies. Make sure you ground your awareness in the changes in breath, circulation including body temperature, and muscle flexibility.

Inverted Postures (handstand, shoulderstand or plow). Psychologically, inverted yogic practices make us feel that our world is turned upside down. The sages have said if we could get used to that feeling, we could adapt to change when it happens without warning.

Parivrtta Trikonasana **(revolved triangle).** Before taking the completed posture, twist from the waist with arms extending out the sides, coming back to center several times until you sense the opening in the lower back and waist. Then take the full posture.

Ardha Baddha Padma Paschimottanasana **(1/2 bound lotus posterior stretch).** Stop when you feel the slightest resistance. Stay at this place until something changes, until you sense a new edge.

Practice off the Mat

Practice being open and receptive to change. Something as simple as changing your hairstyle or wearing different colored clothing can give you a refreshing perspective to the transitions of living.

Look at all the twists and turns in your life. Recognize how life's stages create new opportunities as well as new challenges.

Celebrate the changes of the seasons with a Labor Day party or a Vernal Equinox (March 21) Tea.

Wise Words

Embracing change creates ease and freedom in your world.

The only constant is change.

Notes

Notes

Give yourself room for expansion. Give yourself room to change.

Allow change to happen to you. Don't resist it.

Sunrise and sunset are obvious reminders of change.

May we all learn to accept life's constant changes.

Asanas

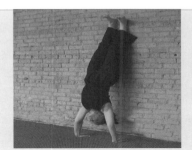

Headstand

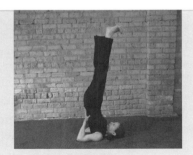

Shoulderstand

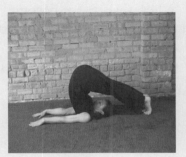

Plow

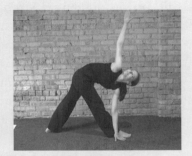

Revolved Triangle

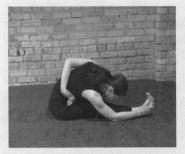

Ardha Baddha Padma Paschimottanasana
half bound lotus posterior stretch

Notes

Fear

Intention: To use the tools of yoga to deal with fear.
Approximate Length: 3 minutes

As terrorism becomes more of a threat to our homeland security, how do we as yogis deal with our own internalized view of fear?

When fear takes over our lives, we are less willing to take risks. This shuts down the third *chakra* — the solar plexus — the center of our will, power and inner strength. When this *chakra* becomes deficient, we tend to close off to life's unlimited potential. Living a fearful existence will most assuredly keep your spirit at bay.

As yogis, we take a very pragmatic view of the world, understanding that fear is recognized as part of human existence. Whether you lived in caves thousands of years ago fearing the attack of a lion, or you live in New York City fearing another 9-11, violence and suffering have always been part of this world.

So what kind of practice should we have if we live in fear of bombings, muggings, or other people? Is there a breathing exercise that helps us through a panic attack? Are there actual tools for this?

Yoga's path itself is the tool for the liberation of suffering. The practice of *asana* and *pranayama* are two of the most powerful tools for releasing the fear, anxiety and the resulting anger that gets locked in the body's tissues.

Our practices today will allow us to reconnect and balance our solar plexus and open the armor that protects the heart center. When these *chakras* are open, we can connect with the priorities of the present moment, of gratitude and of love. Then instead of letting fear lead your day, closing you off from your life, you can fill your heart with lifeforce.

176

Asanas for Deepening

Gentle Backbends. Depending on levels of fear, it may be best to begin with a series of gentle backbends to release the armor around the solar plexus and heart. Backbends stimulate circulation in the spine to make us feel more vital and alive. Almost any backbend can be tamed to nurture this effort: **Unsupported Cobra (no arms), Bridge, Half Locust, Lunge, Standing Backbend (with hands supporting the lower waist).**

Ustrasana **(camel).** Focus on opening the solar plexus and heart center. In the final stages, imagine your heart lifting out of its cage to flourish with love, compassion and inner wisdom. Let *prana* circulate and bring energy to all areas. Camel also helps relieve depression caused by anxiety.

Tittibhasana **(firefly).** Helps balance the third *chakra* and develops courage. Have fun and don't bother with whether you can complete the final pose or not. If you're worried about falling on your face, put a pillow or blanket in front of you.

Practice off the Mat

Anxiety Attacks. Practice 2 to 1 breathing where exhale is approximately twice as long as inhale and follow with 4 to 8 rounds of of *nadi shodhana*.

Imagine that your body is lying on the sands of a warm tropical beach. With your exhalation, feel a wave pass downward through the body, carrying away wastes, fatigue and all worries. With the inhalation, a fresh wave passes upward through the whole body, carrying a feeling of energy and well-being from an ocean of cosmic vitality. Breathe this way 10 times.

Have you been closing off your spirit in an effort to protect it? Meditate on the heart center, where fear can get locked. Imagine that you are holding the key and unlock the gate of the heart, feeling the fear and anxiety escape.

Notes

Notes

By meditating on the heart center, we become attuned to deep-seated emotions and reconnect to life as it really is.

If fear is taking you over, think about the very worst outcome of the situation. What happens? What body sensations do you feel? When you hit rock bottom, you can only go up. By thinking of the worst rather that denying or suppressing the result, we can move through the fear that restricts our lifeforce and keeps us locked in our self-induced prison.

Wise Words

We cannot change the world, only ourselves.

Through mindful practice we develop concentration that leads to strength of mind.

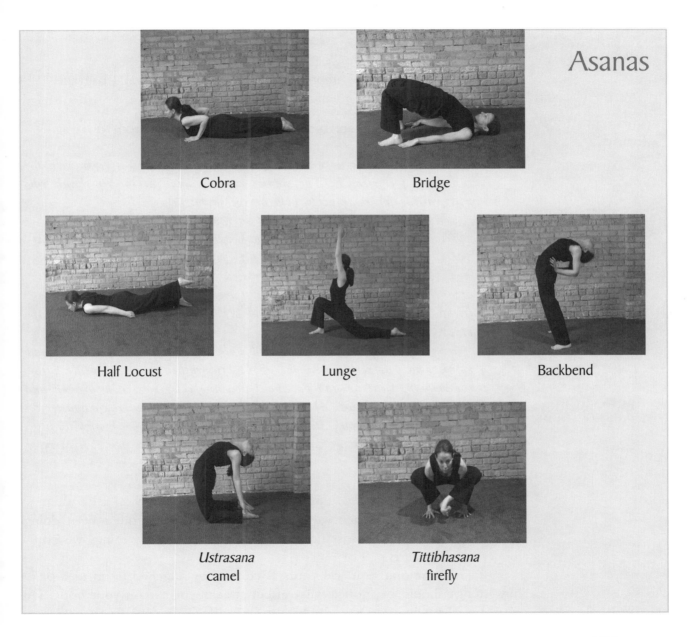

Asanas

Cobra

Bridge

Half Locust

Lunge

Backbend

Ustrasana
camel

Tittibhasana
firefly

Letting Go

Intention: To identify the importance of giving up emotional baggage.
Approximate Length: 3 minutes

How many of us are carrying emotional baggage from years ago? Here's a parable:

Two monks were walking down a road toward a river with the intention of crossing it. The monks saw a woman at the riverbank who was waiting for someone to help her get across.

This was centuries ago and in those days, any contact with women was forbidden. The first monk said to the second monk, "That woman needs help. Shall we take her across the river with us?"

The second monk angrily replied, "We can't do that, we'd be breaking our sacred vows!" The first monk thought about what his friend said, then took the woman on his back and carried her across the river.

After crossing the river and walking a long distance, the second monk who was very distraught about his brother monk's contact with the woman, went on and on about how the vows were now broken and what were they to do? How would they explain this at the monastery?

The first monk stopped, looked at the second monk and said, "Brother, I left that woman two miles back. Why are you still carrying her?"

The *Yama aparigraha,* non-possessiveness, can teach us a lot about letting go of baggage. When we hold onto our own ideas, our way of doing things, and negative circumstances, we hold on to so many things we no longer need to carry.

The next time you feel yourself completely attached to an idea of how things should be, notice what effect attachment has on your body. Do your muscles tighten? Does the breath feel stifled? Is your face tense?

Notes

Notes

Today our intention is the practice of letting go. Think of your yoga mat as a sacred place in which you can bring all of your buried baggage to the surface and give it over to the universe. Only by letting go, forgiving and allowing guilt to fade away can we be in the moment and let life lead us.

Asanas for Deepening

Kurmasana (tortoise). Surrender to the outcome. Let the stretch, breath and open state of mind lead you. Be patient and notice how the mind begins to let go of it's clutches.

Baddha Konasana with Brick (bound angle). Sit in *Baddha Konasana* with a brick between your feet and choose the perfect moment to let go. Don't be in a rush to come out of the pose.

Reclining Twist. Practice the willingness to be present and let things happen.

Practice off the Mat

If you have children, pick your battles. Choose the ones that are most important; let go of everything else.

If you always want to be the driver so that you can be in control, try letting someone else do it for a change.

Do you always have to get the last word in? Try letting someone else do it.

Are you still carrying a grudge over a disagreement with a friend, relative or business associate? Is there someone you haven't spoken to in years? Do you still feel the same guilt, heartbreak, or anger you did when it happened? Is there any reason why you need to carry this burden? Let it go, once and for all. This doesn't necessarily mean you're letting this person back in your life. It simply means you're able to move on.

Notes

Wise Words

Surrender is believing that we have done all that we can and trusting that things will work out.

Letting go means accepting your life without resistance.

When we practice releasing the past, we discover what actually exists within us. This is our authentic self.

Stay centered. Centering teaches us how to be compassionate with ourselves and flexible with our thoughts.

Asanas

Kurmasana
tortoise

Baddha Konasana with brick
bound angle

Reclining Twist with Eagle Legs

Patience

Intention: To practice patience and recognize impatience in our lives and in our yoga practice.

Approximate Length: 4 minutes

It seems that of all the negative emotions we deal with, impatience is the most prominent. We see it in toddlers, business people, parents and seniors. You probably see it in your yoga practice.

Impatience manifests itself in many ways. A friend of mine was waiting at a popular pizza place to pick up her order. It was a very busy Sunday evening with wall-to-wall people waiting for their pizzas. The man next to her was being very impatient. He keep whispering under his breath, "Where's my damn pizza?" Finally, when his name was called, he yelled at the counterman. "This is a disgrace," he shouted, "you said it would be ready by 6 o'clock!" The counterman said apologetically, "I'm sorry you've been waiting so long, sir, but it *is* 6 o'clock." "No it's not!" the man shouted back, "It's 6:05!"

My pizza-less friend laughed at the absurdity of this scenario. Yet, how many of us can honestly say we've *never* been this steamed with impatience?

As a society, we suffer with impatience because our actions are uncontrolled and out of tune with the reality of the now. Our minds are preoccupied with the worries and anxieties of yester-day or tomorrow and it's difficult to involve ourselves in the present. Rather than live in the moment, we find ourselves wanting things to be faster, better, and flow more smoothly. It's as though we're in a cosmic disagreement with how things are really happening. We need to realize that in order to expand our level of patience, we must learn to accommodate the moment.

Our yoga practice provides one of the best and most systematic approaches to regaining our patience. *Asanas* bring us back in touch with the physical body. We begin to feel again. We begin to notice those body sensations of impatience. We learn how to wait and let our bodies open at their own pace.

During today's practice, when impatience-driven anxiety comes up, rather than push these thoughts away, be mindful that they are part of the moment. And like all moments, they will pass.

Patience is a form of wisdom. It shows us that we must accept the fact that things evolve in their own time.

Asanas for Deepening

Over time the body unfolds. If you honor exploration and patience, you discover how everything changes all the time. This is the basis of learning to live in the moment.

Janu Shirshasana **(head-to-knee pose).** Don't rush past the early stages of the stretch wanting to be someone you're not organically ready to be. Find your first place of resistance and adapt before going any further. Once you're settled, bring your attention to where you feel the breath in your body. From that place, follow the movement of each inhalation and exhalation. Notice what comes up. Are you calm? Does the mind wander? Is this a place of clarity for you? When feelings of impatience come up, bring yourself back to the movement of the breath.

Vasisthasana **(side plank).** Take the posture in as many stages as necessary. Try it first with the bottom knee on the floor. Then extend the legs, first practicing balance. Finally, extend the top arm strongly upward.

Child's Pose. Take a deep full breath into the muscles of your back and practice the willingness to be present.

Notes

Practice off the Mat

Next time you're in a restaurant waiting for your order, think about the man and his pizza. Then ask yourself, can I wait five minutes for *my* order?

Do you interrupt others when they're speaking? Do you find your mind moving faster than the speed of light, your words unable to wait? Next time this happens, first become aware of it, then try to pause and really listen to the other person speaking. You may find you're missing half the conversation!

Sometimes the best patience practice is to watch what others do. The man at the pizza place was able to awaken my friend to the impatience in the world. If you have a friend, relative, or co-worker who acts with impatience, spend some time with this person with the intention of looking at his or her impatient characteristics. Without judging or trying to change this person, find out what it is that makes this person impatient. Look at their physical reactions, listen to their tone of voice. Learning to identify others' negative emotions will help you recognize them in yourself. And, if you maintain your sense of the moment with clarity and calm, you'll be setting an excellent example.

The world is full of places to practice patience: traffic jams, the long line at the bank, store, or pizza place, or waiting for someone to e-mail a reply or return your call. As you go through your day, you'll discover dozens of situations in which to practice.

Quick Calm Breath or the Waiting-In-Line Breath. Exhale to a mental count of seven, hold four; inhale to a mental count of four, hold four. Practice four cycles. Adjust your count if breath length feels shallow.

Wise Words

Notes

It's said that much of our discontent with life comes from never fully experiencing it exactly as it happens.

Impatience is a defensive response to a situation that isn't going our way.

When we experience the calmness that results from our yoga practices, we become more centered, satisfied and patient.

Our thoughts can overwhelm our perception of the present moment because the mind is too busy in the future or the past. Impatience arises because things are not moving as fast as our thoughts.

Asanas

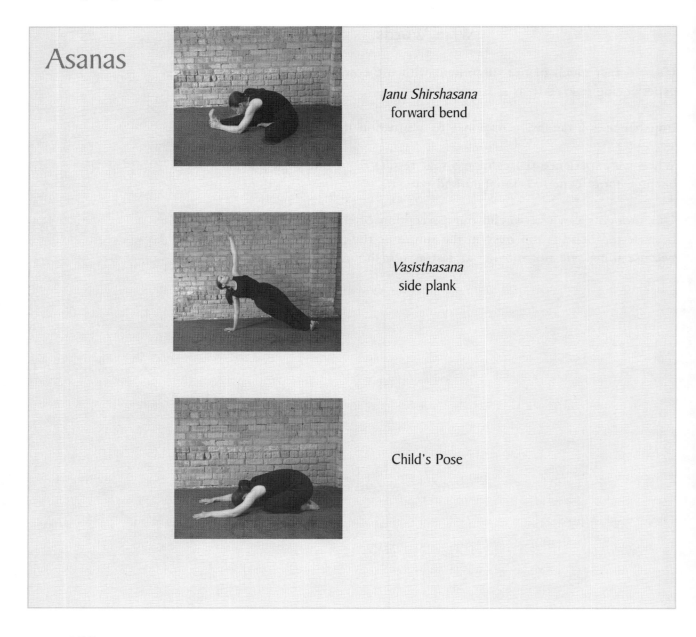

Janu Shirshasana
forward bend

Vasisthasana
side plank

Child's Pose

Chapter Eight

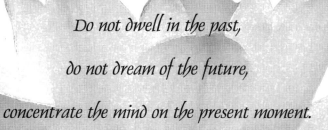

Do not dwell in the past,

do not dream of the future,

concentrate the mind on the present moment.

Buddha

Mindfulness

Have you ever driven somewhere and missed the scenery completely? You did all the driving, but never bothered to look around you.

Think of all the other experiences you miss because you're not paying attention. When you apply mindfulness to your daily activities like driving, brushing your teeth, or eating your morning bowl of cereal, your life becomes a moving meditation.

The lessons that follow will illustrate moving into mindfulness by paying attention.

Once mindfulness is top of mind, you'll be amazed at how much of life you may have missed. As the saying goes, "Those who are awake live in a state of amazement."

Mindfulness:
The Core of Practice

Intention: To integrate mindfulness into practice.
Length: 2 minutes

It's said by many that in order to practice yoga, you don't have to be flexible or strong, you just have to be awake.

Mindfulness is the core of yoga practice. It's what separates our *asana* practice from becoming another stretch. Mindfulness is fully experiencing what happens in the here and now. It's the art of becoming deeply aware of the present instant.

Mindfulness means we're doing one thing at a time. We put our full attention into what we're doing — whether it be our yoga practice, driving the car, or talking to our friends — so we can be awake in that moment.

When we're mindful, we're not missing what's happening now by thinking about the past or future. Our inner focus is in charge; distractions stay on the peripheral of the mind. Our focus stays intact and our immediate experience is fully realized.

The emotional benefits of mindfulness are boundless. It helps us turn down all the noise in our heads — the anger, the doubts, the worries about tomorrow, the clinging to the past.

In our practice, it begins by feeling the pose come to life, sensing the response of the breath, being mindful of stretch, strength, balance and our boundaries.

Lie in *shavasana*. Pay attention to your breath. Let your mind become absorbed in the sound of the inhale and the sound of the exhale. As if you're watching the waves of the ocean, let your mind be naturally drawn into the presence and stillness. The breathing is always changing. There's no single breath the same as the last.

Asanas for Deepening

Practice postures using an internal mantra to help you focus. It could be any set of words that has meaning for you. If you don't have a mantra, use an affirmation such as "I am strong," or "Practice patience." The mantra can be inhaled and exhaled such as "let" on the inhale, "go" on the exhale.

Surya Namaskara (**sun salutation**). When flowing through postures, be mindful of the muscular action, like a full body stocking. Hug your muscles to the bones, draw your energy towards the midline of the body. Try not to miss anything here, not a joint, a muscle or a thought.
Natarajasana (**king dancer**). Breathe smoothly, and bring the pose to life. Support your mindfulness with *prana*. Accept where you are in this moment without striving, without comparing or judging.
Reclining Leg Cradles. When you can't pull the leg in any tighter, stay where you are, maintain the action of the pose and relax with the intensity of the stretch. Close your eyes and let go into who you really are.

Practice off the Mat

Allow mindfulness to seep into your actions when you brush your teeth, wash the dishes, talk on the phone or taste that first sip of morning coffee.

One-Step Meditation. Whenever you feel yourself becoming unfocused or too busy to concentrate, try the one-step meditation. This is a walking meditation that's done walking very slowly, one-step at a time.

Each time you take a step forward, mentally say "one" and as the opposite foot comes forward, say "step." As you do this, take in all that's happening at the moment; how the feet feel on the ground, how the knees bend, how the weight shifts from left to right.

Mindfulness, like all things of merit, can be accomplished one step at a time.

Mindfulness of Breath. Count each set of in and out breaths as one until you reach ten. The object is not to get to ten but to become aware of how much the mind rambles into the past and future and to bring yourself back to the present — the only place where there is truly any control.

Wise Words

Practice mindfulness during your daily living as an approach that encourages you to stop and smell the roses.

Yoga is the method by which the restless mind is calmed and the energy directed into constructive channels.

Be mindful, because this moment will pass and if you're somewhere else, you will not have lived it.

Notes

Asanas

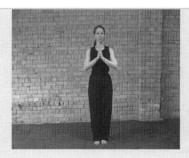

Surya Namaskara
sun salutation
(see p.101 for basic 12 poses)

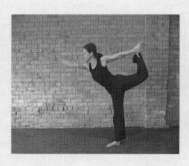

Natarajasana
king dancer

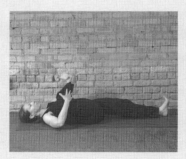

Reclining Leg Cradles

Paying Attention

Intention: To learn objectivity of the mind; to take a step toward meditation.
Approximate Length: 2 minutes

According to yoga philosophy, the world is exactly as it needs to be. This means that everything that happens to us personally and globally, whether we like it or not, is exactly what's supposed to happen. Our mindfulness practice, regardless of whether it's planting tulips or practicing triangle, is about noticing when we're *not* paying attention.

When you begin to notice and pay attention to life as it is, the spiritual questions begin to come up. In the yogic tradition, they can only be worked out through clear thinking.

Our *asana* practice imparts to us the importance of the present; to be in the moment whether we are depressed or anxious or calm or tired. This gives us the means to become aware of *vrittis*, the fluctuations of the mind. We begin by first learning to focus on the gross aspects of the body and then on the more discriminating components of *prana* and our ability to control it.

Gradually, we begin to develop the mind's capacity to focus on one thing — this is called *dharana* — the concentration one needs in order to meditate. From here, the mind instinctively flows into *dhyana* or meditation, the seventh limb of *Raja* Yoga.

Today our intention is the eternal practice of training the mind to pay attention — that is, to wake up to life, both internally and externally.

Asanas for Deepening

In all postures, work with the internal mantra: "Breathing, grounding, lengthening." Exhale, breathing down to the toes, and inhale up to the crown of the head, feeling and sensing the breath move through you. **Inverted Table.** Feel the hands and feet strongly reaching down, spine lengthening in both directions, shoulders open and moving away from each other. Look straight ahead, make your *drishti* (focus point) the tips of the knees, checking to make sure they're tracking straight ahead. *Matsyasana* **(fish).** Chest continues to lift through the pose, lungs are engaged in the awareness of breath, and spine lifts into the back. *Padmasana* **(lotus or half lotus).** Weight of the body sinks into the earth. Awaken the crown of the head and allow it to rise to the heavens. Expand the body, expand the mind. Step away from the thinking process and simply watch what unfolds.

Practice off the Mat

This practice can be done anywhere at anytime and is a highly recommended technique for aspiring meditators.

Sit with eyes closed. Just sit. Focus your attention on your breath, a mantra, or a focus point such as a candle or deity.

What happens? Do you notice a pain in your back? Do you hear your breath? Feel your heart beating? Are you thirsty? Just feel that. Where does the mind go? Are you frustrated? Impatient? Calm? Try to just witness these thoughts and sensations without changing or judging.

See how long you can sit in mindfulness. Now open your eyes and reveal what has just happened. How long were you able to sit before your thoughts clouded the open spaces of your mind? The more you practice, the quicker you can step back from your thoughts and simply be the observer.

Wise Words

Notes

In yoga *asana,* we live from moment to moment in the sensation, we are one with the feeling.

What do we do with our available *prana?* We can devour loads of mental energy by unknowingly allowing thoughts to dangle off to other places and people.

It's through continuous and vigilant practice that we begin to develop the objectivity of the mind.

Asanas

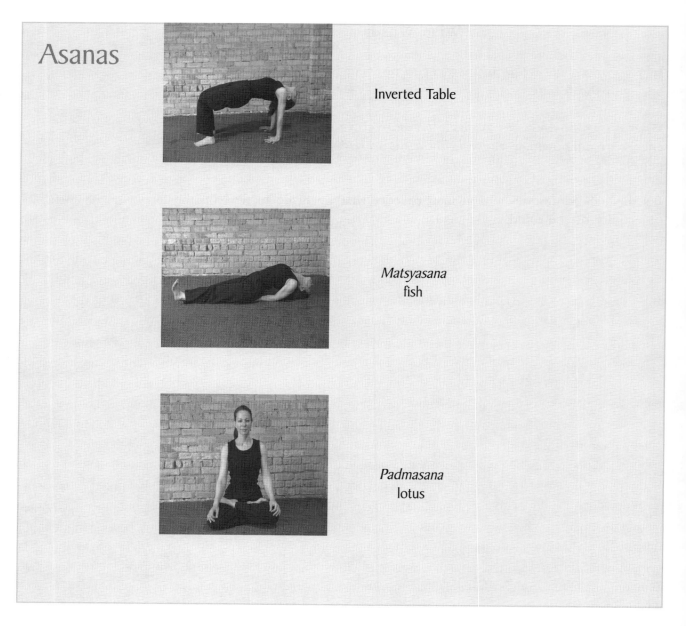

Inverted Table

Matsyasana
fish

Padmasana
lotus

Dharana

Intention: To learn and experience concentration.
Approximate Length: 1 minute

Dharana is the sixth limb of *Raja* Yoga. The objective of this limb is to hold our concentration in one direction. When we apply *dharana,* we light up one particular activity of the mind and the brighter it becomes, the more the other activities of the mind fall away. This practice stops the mind from rambling by willfully holding it on some type of focus point, like a mantra or the breath or a point on the body.

The attention of internal body adjustments in each pose brings awareness to the muscles, joints, and organs. But they also adjust the mind into the present moment. When we consciously drop the shoulders, the mind becomes present. When the mind wanders, the shoulders rise. These adjustments are focus points that tell the mind, be here, not somewhere else.

The technique of *dharana* in *asana* helps us learn and integrate the control of the breath and *prana* within the body. The practice naturally leads to concentration and strength of our emotional body.

Asanas for Deepening

Virabhadrasana **II (warrior II).** The *drishti* (focus point) is the tip of the second finger of the hand you are facing. Keep the *drishti* steady as the awareness of the pose depends on it.
Candle (squat on toes with hands in prayer position over the head). Let go of any exertion and tension and let the legs support you. Flow with whatever may happen and let your mind be focused on your toes.
Upavistha Konasana **(seated angle)**. Release any uneasiness along the

length of your spine. Deepen your awareness, feel for more subtle areas of hold, and use your breath to soften and relax. Here, physical position has little to do with moving toward and into stillness.

Virasana **(hero).** This is a pose of dynamic tranquility and a means to cultivating inner stability. Many use seated hero as a meditation posture. Apply the breath to gently express the meaning of the pose. Exhale and feel the sit bones drop into the earth. Inhale and draw up the front of the spine, lifting the soft tissues at the front of your spine.

Practice off the Mat

Yoga philosophy teaches us that if we want to live a contented existence, we have to break the patterns that keep us running from any discomfort or unpleasantness.

To practice *dharana*, (concentration) become aware of the breath. Place your attention on your abdomen, then let it rest lightly inside on top of the diaphragm muscle. Once you can feel the breath, don't concern yourself with the way you breathe. Instead, let the breath simply move through you as you watch it.

Try not to miss a breath: breathing out, breathing in. If the mind wanders off the path, don't get stuck on a thought and get involved. Instead gently bring your mind back and begin again.

Your only objective is to surrender to the movement of the breath. Let it come, let it go, whatever it is.

Each inhale, each exhale, move it on through.

If you thread this practice into your day, at work, in your car, while sitting in a waiting room, virtually anywhere, you will begin to experience all the benefits of *santosha,* contentment.

Wise Words

Dharana is preparation for *dhyana* (meditation).

When the mind has become purified by yoga practices, we release a great potential for inner healing.

The moment we start to force, we begin to lose awareness of the nervous system or of the situation.

When we lose our concentration, bring the attention back to the object of focus.

During *asana,* frequently ask yourself, "Where am I now? Where is my focus? Can I take it deeper?"

When we really begin listening to our minds, we experience the waterfall of distractions. Simply observe and watch one thought fall into another.

Asanas

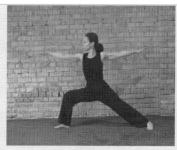

Virabhadrasana II
warrior II

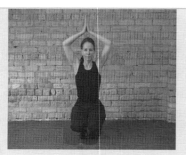

Candle

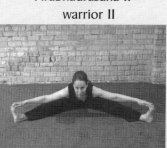

Upavistha Konasana
seated angle

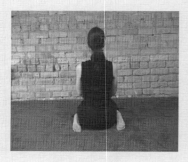

Virasana
hero

Mindfulness of Gratitude

Intention: To live in a state of gratitude.
Approximate Length: 5 minutes

Mindfulness of gratitude is a very powerful practice. Practicing mindfulness of gratitude guides us to an immediate experience of being connected to the realization that there is a larger context in which our life is developing.

A gratitude practice is particularly beneficial for those who are troubled with mild depression or carry feelings of negativity about every situation in their life. Some choose a melancholy existence because they don't know any other way.

Our *asana* practice helps us to focus on appreciating the miracle of the body. Remember, it's important to be grateful for having two legs, two arms, and a brain to boot!

When we make *asana* a daily practice, a natural antidepressant kicks in. With mindful breathing our anxiety levels decrease and our mood becomes lifted. The more we practice, the deeper the relaxation response goes.

Quieting the mind and generating a strong connection with the heart adds regenerative energy and an attitude of gratitude to your entire system.

Today we're going to begin our practice with the **Gratitude of Heart** breath. This is like an adjustment for our feelings; when we focus on gratitude, appreciation, compassion or another positive loving emotion, our heart rhythms immediately shift. Blood pressure normalizes. Stress hormones drop. The immune system gets stronger.

During difficult times, **Gratitude of Heart** breath can help ease depression and anxiety.

203

Notes

The essential step in the **Gratitude of Heart** breath is to energetically send out appreciation or love. Feeling these emotions creates a cascade of biochemical events that nourish the body and mind. Emotionally we feel calm, clear and mentally strong.

This is an exceptional way to begin our *asana* practice, because so much of what we do in our poses requires awareness and opening of the heart center.

First, close your eyes and let the body relax. Shift from the outside world to the inside world and gently bring your attention to the area around your heart, the mid-chest. Put your right hand on your heart. Envision your breath going in and out through the heart center, taking very slow, intentional deep breaths.

Now visualize something that's effortless for you to appreciate: your children, friends, parents, God, your pets. Send them genuine gratitude and love as you breathe through your heart. Really feel the *emotion*, not just the thought.

After you've finished the heart breath, try to hold on to those qualities of appreciation and love as long as you can. This acts as a buffer against recurring stress or anxiety.

Asanas for Deepening

Surya Namaskara **(sun salutation).** Practice with an attitude of gratitude. Think of the eternal sun rising and setting, day after day for millions of years — lighting and warming your environment, supplying the necessary elements to grow food and light up your life. Then bring that sun energy into your heart and let it expand and flow within you. Thank the sun for its life-giving powers as you practice *Surya Namaskara* with this sun prayer:

"O lord of light, the sun, master of warmth and peace, destroyer of all diseases, I bow down to thee. I feel your warmth illuminate my heart. I feel your healing rays enlighten my spirit. Please be merciful unto me, O Supreme Being, and shine your energies on my health."

Reclining *Baddha Konansana* (bound butterfly). Opens the chest, quiets the mind, helps relieve anxiety and stress.

Seated *Yoga Mudra*. Succumb to an attitude of admiration for life as you bend forward, head beneath the heart.

***Bhujangasana* (cobra).** Feel spine opening, collarbone lengthening, and chest expanding in the heart center. Notice the *prana* concentrated in the front and back of the heart. Breathe with compassion and gratitude.

***Chakrasana* (wheel).** Improves circulation, stimulates the nervous system and generates a feeling of well being. Increases energy and counteracts depression.

Practice off the Mat

Gratitude Journal. Every night at bedtime, write down five things you are grateful for. You may want to go with the obvious, your health, your family, or your job. But the entries can be as simple (although just as important) as having running water, clean clothes, or the beauty of a rosebud. Within a week, you'll find your daily gratitude level will heighten, your role in life will be more realistic and your anxiety levels will decrease.

Perspective is powerful medicine!

For an entire day, be the messenger of good news. Every time you speak to someone, let it be of something pleasant or uplifting and make a conscious effort to notice and acknowledge what's good about the day.

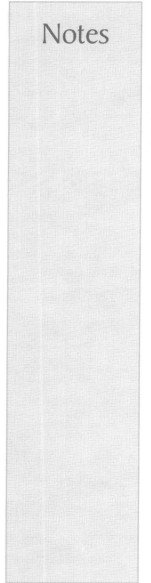

Notes

Wise Words

Every day is a gift, that's why it's called the present.

Living in appreciation makes every day better, and there is always something to appreciate.

May you be awake to the gifts you receive and give.

Asanas

Surya Namaskara
sun salutation
(see p.101 for basic 12 poses)

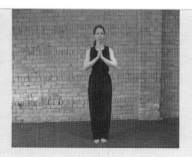

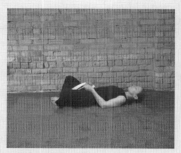

Reclining *Baddha Konasana*
bound butterfly

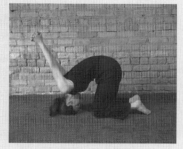

Seated *Yoga Mudra*

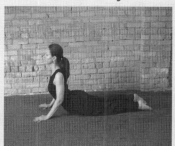

Bhujangasana
cobra

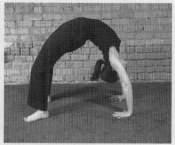

Chakrasana
wheel

Mindful Eating

Intention: To discover awareness and gratitude in eating.
Approximate Length: 2-3 minutes

Do you ever eat, but only taste the first bite? You sit down at the table and put food into your mouth, but your mind is off somewhere else. There's no connection between your mind and your mouth.

When we eat, we are feeding our inner selves. This requires a thoughtful approach because, after all, food sustains life. Eating calmly with full awareness and gratitude feeds the mind and spirit as well as the body.

Most students of yoga find that as the body becomes healthier, we naturally become more sensitive to *what* we eat and *how* we eat. This new awareness helps us make wise choices.

In the yogic point of view, food has properties that influence our physical, mental, emotional and spiritual life. Stale, processed or overripe foods have lost their *prana*. When they're ingested, this leads to a state of dullness and lethargy. Foods with a lot of sugar or caffeine, like chocolate and coffee, over-stimulate and excite the nervous and hormonal systems and counteract the balancing effects of our *asana* practice.

But foods that are as close to the earth as possible, like fresh vegetables, whole grains and fruits, are neither depressing or stimulating. Like our *asana* and *pranayama* practice, they nourish and energize, bringing us into balance and harmony with our bodies, minds and emotions.

It's also important to pay attention to *how much* we eat. *Bhramacharya,* moderation in all aspects of life, is encouraged in yoga. A yogi never comes to a point of complete satiation. Try to fill your stomach with three-quarters food and one-quarter liquid at each meal.

When it comes to your relationship with food, the best advice you can give yourself is to enjoy it. If you devote yourself to the enjoyment and gratitude of the food itself and it's source, you'll find out what truly nourishes you and no longer need what doesn't.

Asanas for Deepening

The *asanas* focus on postures that help food assimilate, digest and eventually move through the system.

***Supta Sukhasana* (reclining easy pose).** This pose is very soothing for heartburn (acid reflux) and improves overall digestion by increasing blood supply to the intestines.

***Marichyasana* (seated twist).** Massages and tones the internal organs and maintains space and mobility in the spine.

Intestinal massage. Sit in **on the heels.** Place fists just above and inside the point of the pelvic bone at the right hip. Bend forward and massage gently up the right side of the abdomen, where the ascending colon is. Continue across the diaphragm (upper abdominal area) to massage the transverse colon, and then down the left side, to complete the process on the descending colon. You should be able to feel (and possibly hear) gas bubbles and blockages being moved along. This massage is excellent for improving elimination problems, including constipation.

***Sarvangasana* (inverted action pose/shoulderstand).** The change in gravity affects the abdominal organs so that the bowels move freely.

Practice off the Mat

Mindful Eating Practice. Start by eating a small piece of food, like a raisin or a piece of popcorn as slowly as possible. Savor the touch and taste of each morsel as you enjoy the sensation of food with total mindfulness. Enjoy the flavors, colors and textures of your meal.

Notes

Notes

Eat alone without any distractions such as the television or newspaper. Simply sit, just you and your food, being mindful of the nourishment your body is receiving.

Invite friends over for a silent mindfulness dinner. Again, no distractions like music, television or reading materials. This is especially interesting when you're eating crunchy foods like cereals or chips, or slurpy foods like stews and soups. Another twist on this technique is to eat in the dark.

Just for fun, try eating with the opposite hand or eating with chopsticks.

Wise Words

Take a moment before you eat quietly to give thanks, reflecting on the food's source and its purpose in your life.

What is your food doing to you? Is it nourishing you? Is it stimulating you or making you sleepy? Can you judge when you're full, or do you overeat until you're stuffed?

Practicing mindfulness in *asana* teaches us to recognize the feeling of fullness.

Pay attention to what you are eating, notice the effect of food in your life and enjoy it as a gift.

Asanas

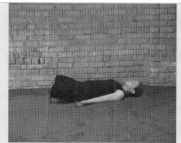

Supta Sukhasana
reclining easy pose

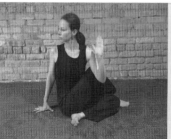
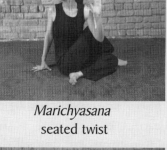

Marichyasana
seated twist

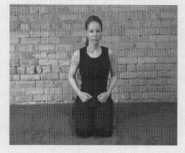

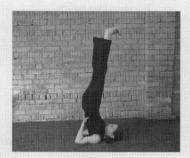

Intestinal Massage

Inverted Action Pose

Sarvangasana
shoulderstand

Setting an Intention

Intention: To create a meaningful objective to *Hatha* Yoga practice.
Approximate Length: 1 minute

When we set our intentions for practice, we let self-observation be our first step. To set an intention requires a certain awareness that we know something about our current situation and ourselves. An intention can be quite simple, such as, "I need relief in the right side of my neck" or "I've been working all day and I want to clear my head." Or your intention may be more complex, such as, "I want to move out of a bad relationship" or, "I want to work on a very challenging posture to develop my self-confidence."

Keep the intention concrete. Be specific. This will help you maintain focus in your practice. Witness yourself in complete mindfulness before beginning, before the first conscious breath.

Asanas for Deepening

Rocking Chair. Wakes up the energy in the spine.
Arm Stretch. Sit in any seated posture. Stretch the arms out to the sides. Let the movement be carried by some deep inner energy rather than just muscle power. Think of a loved one you're trying to stretch out to. Notice how intention matters.
Inverted Plank. Relax into the full expression of the pose as you observe the responses and fluctuations between outer body, will and ego.
Hidden Lotus. Take *Padmasana* **(lotus)** onto the knees, then slowly walk your hands forward until the abdomen is on the ground.
Vinyasa. **Child's Pose** to **Downdog** to **Updog** to **Child's Pose**. Move with the breath. Think only of the synchronicity of the breath, not of the

movement itself. If the breath is restricted in any way, consciousness will also be restricted.

Practice off the Mat

During your day, set your intention for doing what you need to do. Bring your mind to the intention with full acceptance in the moment. Be sure to breathe in compassion for yourself, especially if it's something you don't enjoy doing, such as running errands. Breathe self-acceptance into your eyes, your skin, muscles, bones and heart. Breathe and receive.

Wise Words

Before you begin to move your body, pause to observe how you feel. Notice your physical sensations, the quality of your natural breath and your state of mind.

You can practice the same pose every day for ten years, and by applying mindful intention, have a different experience every time you practice it.

Notes

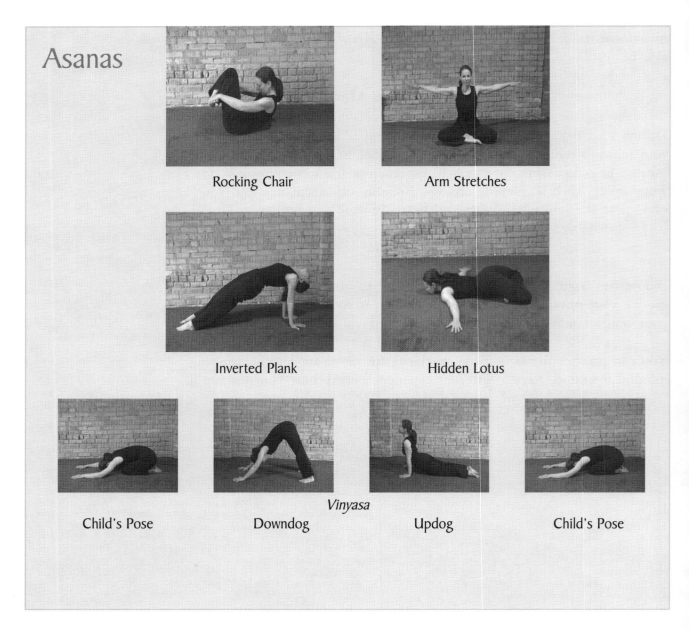

Asanas

Rocking Chair

Arm Stretches

Inverted Plank

Hidden Lotus

Child's Pose

Downdog

Vinyasa

Updog

Child's Pose

Chapter Nine

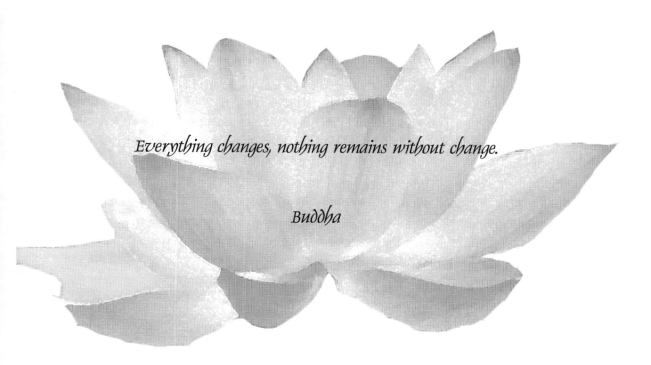

Everything changes, nothing remains without change.

Buddha

The *Chakras*

The *chakras* are the seven major energy centers that regulate the flow of subtle energy in our bodies. They're arranged vertically from the base of the spine to the top of the head.

Chakra is the Sanskrit word for wheel. These "wheels" are spinning vortexes of energy. As centers of lifeforce consciousness, *chakras* are the prominent areas where we take in and disburse life energies. Through external and internal life situations, a *chakra* can either be lacking or have too much energy and therefore, become imbalanced.

The lessons that follow introduce each *chakra*, their characteristics, and their balances and imbalances. Learning about them gives us insight into our inner and outer worlds so we can enjoy each *chakra*'s positive experiences and reverse their negatives ones. The lessons are intended to awaken and balance these centers of consciousness to facilitate healing and help us live a more fulfilling and meaningful life.

The *Chakras*

Chakra **One**: *Muladhara* – root

Chakra **Two**: *Svadhisthana* – lower abdomen/pelvis

Chakra **Three**: *Manipura* – solar plexus

Chakra **Four:** *Anahata* – heart center

Chakra **Five:** *Visuddh*a – throat center

Chakra **Six:** *Ajna* – eyebrow center

Chakra **Seven:** *Sahasrara* – crown center

Root *Chakra*
Muladhara

Intention: To awaken and balance the root *chakra*.
Approximate Length: 2 minutes

The first *chakra* or root *chakra* is called *muladhara*. This is the building block on which all the other *chakras* rest. It's located at the perineum, midway between the anus and the genitals, and it relates to the element of earth and vibrates to the color red.

The main consideration in the root *chakra* is survival. Only when our survival needs are met can we feel grounded and safe in our lives. If this *chakra* is unbalanced any growth will be without roots. Therefore it will lack the stability necessary for long term change.

When this *chakra* is balanced, we have good physical energy and health and a sense of groundedness. We feel comfortable in our bodies, and we feel a sense of safety and security.

When this *chakra* is extreme, having too much root, we have a feeling of heaviness, we're slow moving, we tend to overeat so we're sluggish, and we have a resistance to change.

If this *chakra* is lacking energies, we feel spacey, insecure, fearful, and anxious and have a tendency to be underweight.

Our physical imbalance manifests as aches and pains in the legs, feet and bones. A person with an excessive first *chakra* may experience constipation; a person with whose first *chakra* is lacking energy may experience diarrhea.

Today our practice will focus on noticing gravity, and moving very slowly and deeply to feel all aspects of the body and it's roots in the earth.

Notes

217

Asanas for Deepening

Foot Stomping. Stamp the feet to open the foot *chakra*s.
Emphasize Standing Poses. Standing postures help open and strengthen the lower body and root attention downward.
Chant *lam* (seed sound of *muladhara*) with movement. Combine *Uttanasana* with the seed sound *lam* (pronounced "lum") as you exhale down to the earth. Bend the knees if fingertips don't touch the ground. Repeat 3-6 times.
Asvini Mudra. Begin with *Makarasana* **(crocodile)** with legs together. Exhale and contract the buttocks and pull in the anal sphincter muscles. Inhale and relax completely. This helps strengthen and energize the muscles around the base of the spine and pelvic floor, and brings awareness to the root.
Mula Bhanda **(root lock).** A prolonged contraction of the muscles at the perineum. The contraction changes the flow of subtle energy (*prana*) in the body by reversing the downward moving energy in the root *chakra*, causing it to move upward. Holding energy here is stabilizing and calming and enhances concentration.

Practice off the Mat

To increase first *chakra* energy, eat proteins and earthy foods like root vegetables. Spend time outdoors: go bike riding, power walking, or try gardening. Tune into your body.

To decrease root *chakra* energy, lighten up: eat organic, fresh and whole foods as opposed to processed, sleep less and increase the movements of the body.

Wise Words

Muladhara means support or foundation.

We can only truly share in and value our life experiences when we are first able to meet our most basic survival issues of safety and security.

When *muladhara chakra* is healthy and balanced, we feel nurtured and experience our connection to the whole.

Notes

Asanas

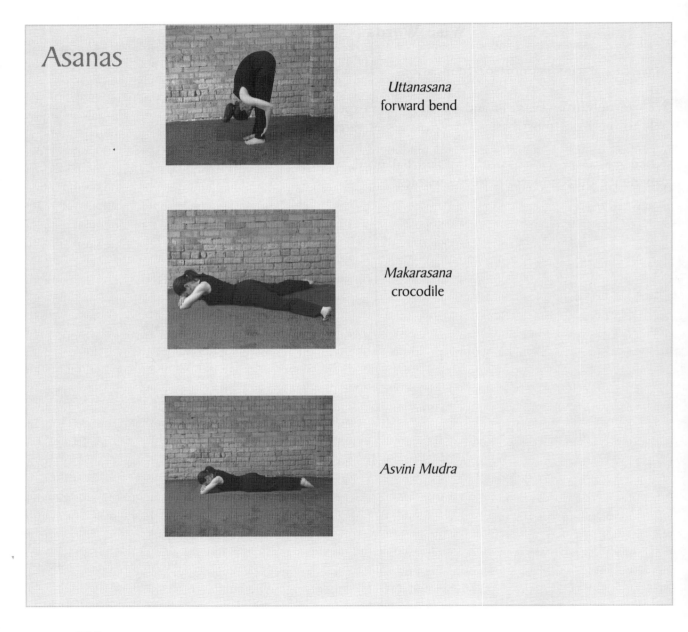

Uttanasana
forward bend

Makarasana
crocodile

Asvini Mudra

Pelvic *Chakra* *Svadhisthana*

Intention: To awaken and work through imbalances in the second *chakra*.
Approximate Length: 4 minutes

The second *chakra*, or *svadhisthana*, is located at the lower abdomen or pelvis and corresponds to the sacral vertebrae. This area links into the sciatic nerve and is the center of motion for the body.

It relates to the element of water and vibrates to the color orange. Our motivating principle in *chakra* two is pleasure. Once survival needs are met in *chakra* one, we turn toward enjoyment.

When this *chakra* is balanced, we experience happiness, joy and sensuality. We have a passion for life, we're expressive, trusting and sexually satisfied.

Imbalance of this *chakra* causes feelings of guilt, powerlessness, insecurity, isolation and over-sensitivity. There's usually blaming of the self and of others, emotional instability, and manipulative behavior.

When this *chakra* is overactive, we may have sexual addictions, obsessive attachments, crave stimulation and be excessively sensitive.

When this *chakra* is lacking, we may feel fearful of change, have poor social skills, be stiff in the body and in life, and have guilty feelings.

Physical symptoms of imbalance manifest in the sex organs, large intestines, pelvis, hips, and bladder. Some common physical manifestations of imbalance are impotence, frigidity, infertility and lower back pain.

Today, our practice for opening and balancing the second *chakra* involves working with movement in the hips and lower abdomen. When we're practicing, keep in mind the balanced second *chakra*: experience the joy and pleasure in the body and in life. Move fluidly like water, being sensitive to sensation.

Asanas for Deepening

Standing Pelvic Tilts. Connect with earth energy through the feet and legs and move it into the second *chakra*. Tilt the pelvis forward as you push against the earth. Imagine the energy you're building in the legs is flowing like water into your sacral area.

***Baddha Konasana* Bends with Chant (butterfly with forward bend).** Combine butterfly forward bends with the second *chakra* seed sound *vam* (pronounced "vum") as you exhale and hold the posture. Repeat 3-6 times. As you bend forward, bring awareness to the pleasure center.

Pelvic Rotations with *Bhastrika* Breath (bellows breath). In a seated position, make clockwise pelvic rotations and begin the *bhastrika* breath. Visualize stirring up the life force in this *chakra*. Be sure to rotate in the opposite direction.

Reclining *Virasana* (hero). Relax and tune into a vibrant orange pulsation within the lower abdomen. Allow it to gently open.

Practice off the Mat

Drink Water. In order to unleash stuck energy, we have to be able to move and change. This is the principal purpose of the second *chakra* — to move energy along.

Movement. Walk, dance, run, stretch. Go with the flow of your body.

Rediscover Your Sexuality. Fill your sexual journey with passion and romance. Allow it to be more than just the sexual act; honor the divine within your partner.

Wise Words

Notes

Svadhisthana means "abode of the vital force" or "dwelling place of the self."

A healthy second *chakra* connects us to others without losing our identity.

The desire of this *chakra* is to create and expand without limitation.

Asanas

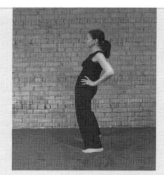
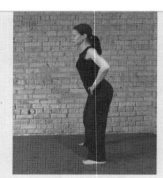

Standing Pelvic Tilts

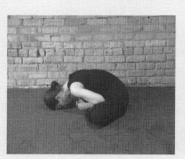

Baddha Konasana
with forward bend

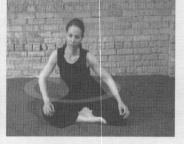

Pelvic roataions
with *Bhastrika* Breath

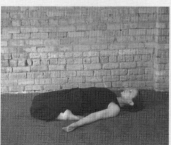

Reclining *Virasana*
reclining hero

Solar Plexus *Chakra*
Manipura

Intention: To awaken and balance the third *chakra*.
Approximate Length: 3 minutes

The third *chakra, manipura,* is located at the solar plexus where the body's energy battery is stored. As *prana* rises up from the first and second *chakras,* it has the potential to become a powerful force in our lives. This *chakra* is associated with the element of fire and vibrates to the color yellow.

Within this *chakra* we develop strength, will and courage. While the second *chakra* may get you moving to make positive changes like quitting smoking or changing jobs, it's the force from the third *chakra* that enables us to move through the excursion.

The intensity of the solar plexus is involved in our self-esteem, courage and the power of transformation.

When this *chakra* is balanced, we're able to make lasting changes, to take risks, and feel a sense of inner power and self-confidence.

When this *chakra* is lacking, we have little energy, bad digestion, low-self esteem and often feel intimidated.

If this *chakra* is extreme, we're controlling, competitive, stubborn and bear too much emphasis on power and social status.

Ulcers, chronic fatigue and digestive problems are common third *chakra* ailments.

Today our practice for opening and balancing the *manipura chakra* embraces poses that fan the flames of the inner fire. In an effort to support this *chakra* on its dynamic journey, it is important for the body's center of gravity to have good muscle tone. This supports our posture, and promotes a sense of will and determination. Having good muscle tone in the abdomen also enhances all the yoga postures and strengthens every system in the body.

Our inner focus is moving with will and purpose, energizing limbs and torso, and building and storing *prana.*

Asanas for Deepening

Navasana (seated boat). Hold the posture for 5 to 10 breaths. Repeat 3-5 times.

Paschimottanasana (posterior stretch) with Chant *ram. Ram* (pronounced "rum") is the seed sound of the third *chakra.* As you exhale into posterior stretch, audibly say *ram.* Hold your awareness at the navel through your exhale. Repeat 3 times.

Standing Strength and Stamina Flow. This series warms the body and builds strength in the abdomen one side at a time. Feel the warrior energy and move from the navel center in all postures. Take 5 breaths in each *asana,* then move to the next.

1) *Tadasana* (mountain)
2) *Virabhadrasana I* (warrior I)
3) *Parshvottanasana* (angle)
4) *Virabhadrasana II* (warrior II)
5) *Trikonasana* (triangle)
6) *Parshvakonasana* (triangle II)
7) *Adho Mukha Shvanasana* (downdog)
8) *Tadasana*

Repeat on the opposite side.

Uddiyana Bandha. Takes energy from the second *chakra* and moves it up to the third for the purpose of purification and detoxifying the system. From a standing position, bend forward and rest your hands just above

Notes

your knees. Exhale completely, pulling your belly back toward the spine. Apply *mula bandha* (root lock). Lift the lower abdomen upward under the rib cavity so navel center will appear concave. Drop the chin toward the chest. Hold. When you need to inhale, lift the chin, release the belly and *mula bandha*. Repeat 2 times.

Practice off the Mat

Risk It. Move beyond what feels safe. Gently push yourself into something new. Start small: for some, taking a risk may be asking the waiter for more mayonnaise. For others, it's buying a house. Weigh the risk in relation to what seems appropriate for the health of your third *chakra*.

Daily Goals. Make a list of daily goals and use your will to accomplish each one. Start small. One item might be to simply make your bed each morning.

Wise Words

Manipura means, "jewel of the lotus" or "lustrous gem."

A balanced third *chakra* connects us with our internal power source and our body's energy battery.

Asanas

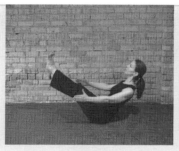

Navasana
boat

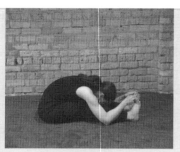

Paschimottanasana
posterior stretch

Standing Strength and Stamina Flow

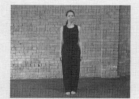

Tadasana
mountain

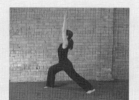

Virabhadrasana
warrior I

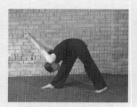

Parshvottanasana
angle

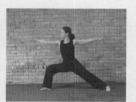

Virbhadrasana II
warrior II

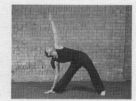

Trikonasana
triangle

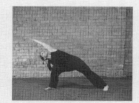

Parshvakonasana II
triangle II

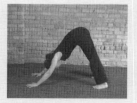

Adho Mukha Shvanasana
downdog

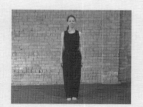

Tadasana
mountain

Heart Center
Anahata

Intention: To awaken and balance the heart center.
Approximate Length: 3 minutes

The fourth *chakra, anahata* or heart center, is the center of the *chakra* system. Its physical location is the heart, lungs, thymus gland, upper chest, upper back, shoulders, arms and hands. The heart *chakra* vibrates to the color emerald green and its element is air, which spreads and energizes.

This *chakra* is the balance point between the lower three *chakra*s and the upper three *chakra*s. It lies halfway between Mother Earth — our connection to the physical plane and Father Sky — our connection to the spiritual plane. The heart center integrates the two.

This *chakra* carries the seed of inner peace and harmony, and as the center expands, the seed opens and grows. When this *chakra* is balanced, we are better able to give and receive love. We are caring, compassionate, accepting and have a peaceful spirit.

When the heart is lacking, we have feelings of shyness and loneliness, an inability to forgive and a lack of empathy. We tend to be critical, intolerant and resentful.

If you notice that your shoulders are rounded inward and your heart sunken, it may be difficult to feel the physical movement that enables this emotional journey to begin.

Symptoms of an overactive *chakra* include co-dependency, jealousy and possessiveness. We've all known people who were jealous of our friends or relatives and feel a certain ownership of the relationship.

Physical imbalances manifest as shallow breathing, asthma, high blood pressure and heart disease.

Notes

Our yoga practices for opening the heart *chakra* involve working with the supporting anatomy around the heart to give the chest some breathing room.

Our internal focus is on releasing blocked or over-flooded emotion. We'll lead with the heart center, working from the heart, not the head.

Asanas for Deepening

Breathing *Bhujangasana* (cobra). Breath in and out of the pose. Open to sensation with each inhale, maintaining that opening as you release to the floor with each exhale.

***Dhanurasana* (bow).** The heart center naturally desires to release and let go. Doing back bends develops the physical opening and surrender which is needed to open the heart completely.

***Trikonasana* (triangle).** Lovingly referred to as the posture of joy because of its heart-opening capabilities. Make sure to spread the wings of the shoulders and feel the heart's backdoor expand between the blades.

Heart-Opening *Vinyasa*. Emphasis is on broadening the shoulders, opening the chest, lifting the sternum and expanding the supporting anatomy around the heart. Hold each position for five breaths.

1) **Easy pose with side stretch**
2) **Easy pose twist**
3) **Seated *Yoga Mudra*.** Hands interlaced behind back, bring forehead to ground.
4) **Downdog/updog/downdog**
5) **Standing *Yoga Mudra***
6) ***Tadasana* (mountain)** with hands in *namaste*. Tune into the rhythm of the heartbeat.

The Heart Connection. *Anahata* governs the sense of touch and rules the hands. Bring hands together in *namaste* (*anjali mudra*) and experience the sensation of hand touching hand. This completes the energy circuit between the hands and the heart and harmonizes the two hemispheres of the brain. Focus the awareness on *anahata chakra*. Silently chant the seed sound of the heart, *yam* (pronounced "yum") with exhale. Feel the vibration gently stirring the heart center.

Practice off the Mat

Practice Gratitude. Gratitude invites the heart to open. Realize how much we have to be thankful for. Thank your loved ones, neighbors, and co-workers. Keep a gratitude journal.

Give of Yourself. Call someone who is lonely, spend time with others who need companionship, do a favor for someone without expecting anything in return.

Forgive. Forgiveness is essential for a healthy heart *chakra*; it frees the heart so energy can move forward. Forgiveness doesn't mean you forget, or even that you have to *involve* the other person. It's simply a method to accept the past, get on with your life and get your heart energy moving.

Wise Words

When fear or depression sets into our bodies, the body contracts in an effort to defend itself.

The heart *chakra* connects the heart to our hands. What the hands are engaged in directly impacts the heart, and what the heart feels impacts the hands.

Notes

231

Notes

Anahata means unstuck, fresh, clean, unhurt.

When the heart is balanced, we're open to the vibrations of universal love.

The lifeforce of the heart connects us to a higher spiritual power, our own heart and the hearts of others.

Asanas

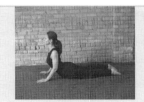

Bhujangasana
cobra

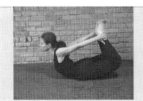

Dhanurasana
bow

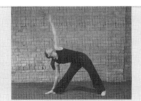

Trikonasana
triangle

Heart Opening *Vinyasa*

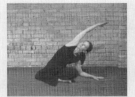

Easy Pose
with Side Stretch

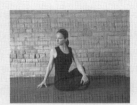

Easy Pose Twist

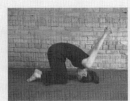

Seated *Yoga Mudra*

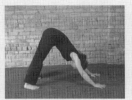

Downdog

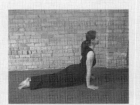

Updog

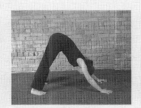

Downdog

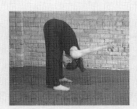

Standing *Yoga Mudra*

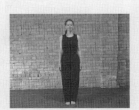

Tadasana

233

Throat Center
Visuddha

Intention: To identify and balance the throat center *chakra*.
Approximate Length: 2 minutes

The throat center and fifth *chakra*, *visuddha*, is the first *chakra* primarily focused on the spiritual plane. It is associated with the color blue and the element of sound.

Vibration, rhythm, music, voice, words and communication are associated with this center. The rhythm of music, expression of dance, singing, and the communication through writing and speaking are all fifth *chakra* ways to express ourselves.

When this *chakra* is balanced, we become aware of the world on a vibrational level, feeling in-tune with our surroundings. The voice is full, listening skills are good and there aren't many "mis-communications."

Physical imbalances may manifest as neck stiffness, teeth grinding, jaw disorders, throat ailments and an underactive or overactive thyroid.

When this energy is lacking in the throat, we have difficulty putting feelings into words, a fear of speaking, speak in a soft voice and often have secrets.

Those with an overactive throat center tend to talk too much and too loud, gossip, criticize and have an inability to listen.

Our *asana* practice for opening this *chakra* includes moving with sound, letting sound move the body, and using sound to release blockages.

Asanas for Deepening

Hum in *asana*. Select any posture such as standing side bend or *Parshvottanasana* (angle) and *hum,* the seed sound of the throat *chakra* on each exhale.

Neck Rolls. Turn head side-to-side and ear to shoulder, using the seed sound *hum* on the exhale.

Halasana **(plow)**. Extend from buttocks to heels. Relax the brain. Keep an opening between your chin and the sternum. Helps stimulate the thyroid gland.

Bhramari **Breath** *pranayama* — The sound of the bumble bee. Clears the mind and soothes the nervous system. Stimulates the throat center. Simulates drone of a bumblebee on the exhale.

Practice off the Mat

Listening. For one day, *really* listen to the people around you. Give others your full attention when they speak to you and show interest and enthusiasm in what they are saying. And don't interrupt!

No Complaints. Avoid criticizing anyone or complaining about anything for one day. This especially includes criticizing yourself. Enjoy the freedom from negative energies.

Peppermint. Add one drop of peppermint essential oil to a glass of water to help open up expression. The peppermint cleanses the throat of mucus and clears away all psychic debris.

Mantra Meditation. Mantra is a tool of the mind that protects us from the traps of non-productive thought and action. The rhythm of the sound works on a subconscious level and penetrates our conscious thoughts by affecting *their* rhythm.

If you don't have a mantra, take a moment to sit quietly each day and say a daily affirmation to yourself. It can be a personal goal or a wish for a loved one. When you say it every day, it becomes a part of you. If you believe this affirmation, you'll become connected to it and it to you.

Notes

Notes

Wise Words

Visuddha means purification. The release of sound purifies and organizes the energy body for entry into higher consciousness.

Sound as a vibration is purifying. Sound affects the cellular structure of matter.

The gift of the throat *chakra* is to be heard, to be understood and to receive truth.

Asanas

Parshvottanasana
angle

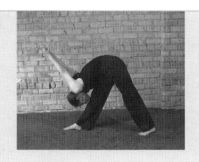

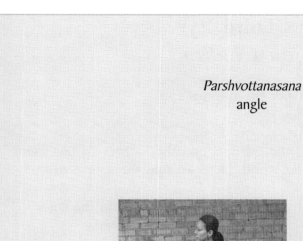 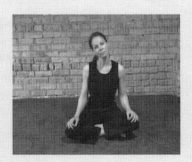

Neck Rolls

Halasana
plow

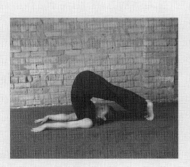

237

The Third Eye
Ajna Chakra

Intention: To awaken and balance the spiritual eye.
Approximate Length: 3 minutes

In the sixth *chakra*, *ajna,* the spiritual eye, the journey of consciousness moves deeper into our inner world. Here we find the source of our inner light.

This center is associated with the element of light and the color indigo. It is located in between and just above the physical eyes.

The sixth *chakra* is the home of intuition, dreams and visions. As children, this *chakra* is open and active. Colors are more vivid. We have imaginary playmates, see dragons, witches and castles. But as we get older, the world around us forces this energy center to close.

As adults, we have to reconnect with this inner window by looking beyond the material world. These internal visual attributes include clairvoyance, telepathy, intuition, dreaming and visualization.

When this *chakra* is balanced, intuition, memory, creativity and dream recall are strong.

When this *chakra* is overactive, we may experience difficulty concentrating, headaches, hallucinations and nightmares.

If this *chakra* is closed, memory is poor, visualization capabilities lacking, we may have an inability to see alternatives and we tend to be skeptical.

Our *asana* focus today is on first inviting stillness and openness into our inner window, and then imagining the energy from the lower *chakra*s moving up into the spiritual eye.

Asanas for Deepening

Practice with Closed Eyes. Keeping the eyes closed during an entire class gives us a fresh perspective on the postures and their healing qualities. Because the eyes provide approximately 85% of our sensory input, students can't be distracted by the room, by other students, or by looking critically at their own bodies.

Matsyasana **(fish).** Puts the focus directly on the third eye.

Earth to Eye Squat. In squat position, bring hands to the front of the body on the ground. Inhale. Exhale and move forehead to the ground as energy moves into the third eye. Repeat 8 times.

Eye Exercises. Do each variation 3 times. There are several methods: 1) Look center, up, center, down. 2) Move eyes clockwise in a circle, then counterclockwise. 3) Focus the gaze on something far such as a tree out the window, and then move the gaze to an object that's visually close, such as the tip of the finger.

Child's Pose Triangle. Place hands on the floor under the forehead, thumbs touching and index fingers touching to make a triangle where the third eye is. Breathe lifeforce into the spiritual triangle.

Padmasana **(lotus).** Chant *om* (seed sound of the spiritual eye) with each exhalation. Rest awareness at the eyebrow center, visualizing energy moving up and down along the subtle channel between the root and eyebrows.

Practice off the Mat

Light Up Your Life. Light is stimulating to consciousness and wakes us up. Start by lighting up your home. Add lamps, open drapes, buy more mirrors, and light candles to shed some light on your third eye.

Notes

Notes

Keep a Dream Journal. Buy a dream interpretation dictionary and record your dreams. Even if you can only remember bits and pieces, dreams reveal the dynamics of our subconscious.

Apply Tiger Balm to the third eye. This helps bring heat and physical awareness to the eyebrow center.

Wise Words

Ajna means command, perception, knowledge and authority.

The *ajna chakra* is the window to the soul.

Clairvoyance is not just for the gifted few. We all have the ability to see clearly if we look deeper and trust our instincts.

Asanas

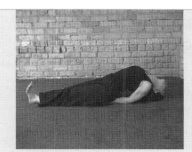

Matsyasana
fish

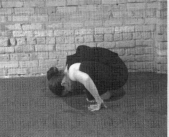

Earth to Eye Squat

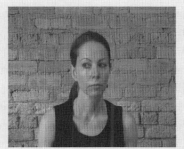

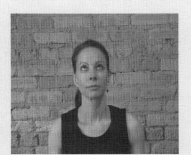

Eye Exercises

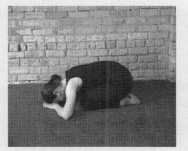

Child's Pose with
Spiritual Triangle

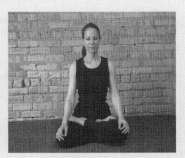

Padmasana
lotus

Crown *Chakra*
Sahasrara

Intention: To awaken and balance the crown *chakra*.
Approximate Length: 2 minutes

The seventh *chakra, sahasrara,* is located at the top of the head and serves as the crown of the *chakra* system, symbolizing the seat of enlightenment.

The element of the seventh *chakra* is thought, corresponding with the highest functions of the mind. It vibrates to the color violet.

Development of the other *chakras* from the root *chakra* upward is a prerequisite for the goal of moving energy up to the crown. Here we are open to divine intelligence, wisdom and understanding. We feel a oneness with a higher power, knowing there is no separation between it and us.

When the crown *chakra* is balanced, we feel at peace with ourselves, have an inner wisdom, a spiritual connection and are open-minded.

When this *chakra* is overactive, one may live in their head or have feelings of being a spiritual elitist, and have a disassociation from the body.

If the crown center is lacking energy, one may be a spiritual cynic or skeptic, have difficulty thinking, a closed mind or rigid belief systems.

Our *asana* practice today for opening and balancing this *chakra* is to focus on awareness of awareness. Witness consciousness, releasing attachments, and connecting to a higher power.

Asanas for Deepening

Uttanasana (standing forward bend)
Chakrasana (wheel)
Handstand Against the Wall (feet against the wall)

Shirshasana (headstand or tripod)
Pranayama: nadi shodhana (alternate nostril)
Padmasana (lotus). Chant *om* with each exhalation. Rest awareness at crown center, visualizing energy moving up and down an imaginary channel between the root and the crown.

Practice off the Mat

Honor the Divine. Visualize your concept of divine spirit, whether its God, angels, Jesus or Buddha. Set aside time each day for spiritual practice and prayer. Look outside and honor the wonder of nature.

Dhyana (**meditation**). The seventh limb in *Raja* Yoga, meditation, is the optimal yogic practice for bringing this *chakra* into balance. Meditation connects us to divine energy and expanded consciousness, and empowers the mind to become more present, clear and insightful. Just as *asana* has been called dental floss for the body, meditation is mental floss for the mind.

Wise Words

Sahasrara means "thousand petal lotus."

The purpose of opening and balancing the crown center is to tune into and surrender to divine consciousness.

Those who are enlightened know the unknown and experience the transcendental meaning of life.

Notes

243

Asanas

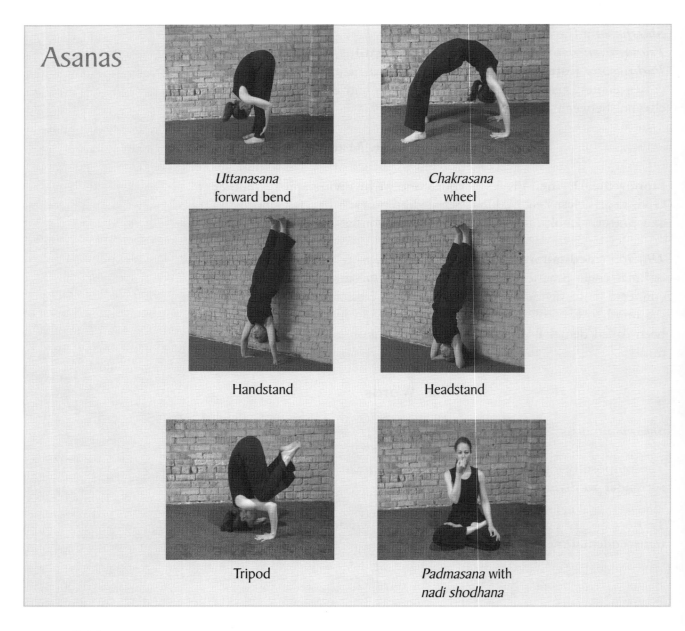

Uttanasana
forward bend

Chakrasana
wheel

Handstand

Headstand

Tripod

Padmasana with
nadi shodhana

Chapter Ten

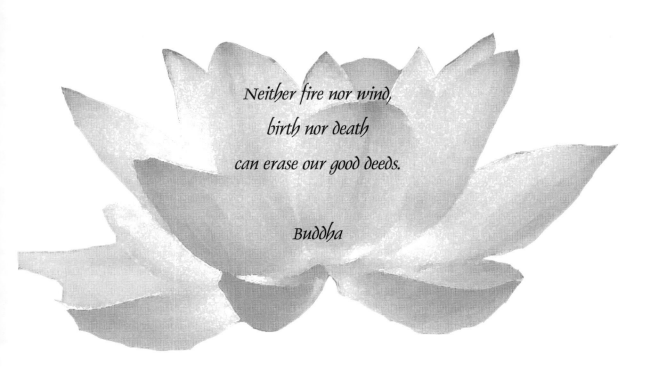

Neither fire nor wind,
birth nor death
can erase our good deeds.

Buddha

Popular Class Beginnings

Sometimes our lessons for the week are just a sprinkling of cosmic seeds that may not fall into any specific yoga category. But their energies are strong and powerful enough get us to think about how we live, what we choose to think and what kinds of things are important to us.

Share the words of these lessons and you may just change someone's day.

Holiday Gratitude

(Recommended for use during Thanksgiving or holiday classes)

Intention: To feel gratitude in the heart.
Approximate Length: 4 minutes

At this time of year, we're taught to count our blessings and be grateful. But gratitude, like everything else, is a *choice*. When we choose to be grateful, we focus on all the things that are right in our life as opposed to the things that are not, such as what we can and cannot do physically in our *asana* practice. Applying this definition to gratitude, we begin to see our entire existence as a miracle rather than just the passing of time.

The practice of gratitude is empowering. It can change the way you perceive your life.

Close your eyes, bring your hands in *anjali mudra (namaste)* and gently give your attention to the center of your chest, the heart center. Focus on the rising and falling of the chest as you breathe in and out. Think about the things in your life that fill you with happiness and joy: your friends, family, pets, whatever fills you with gratitude. As you focus on these things, you may begin to feel warm and calm and content. You are now in a state of gratitude.

Today, let's combine the powerful healing energies of *asana* with the practice of kindness, compassion and gratitude. If you wish, send these healing energies to someone who needs it today.

The Only Constant Is Change

Intention: To illustrate the fact that nothing lasts forever.
Approximate length: 3 minutes

The present situation can change in an instant. The yogi stays tranquil and accepts life's frequent turn of events knowing pleasure, pain, good and bad never last forever.

Here's a parable that shows how quickly life can turn around:

There once was a farmer who had a magnificent prize-winning stallion. The farmer planned to sell him to a wealthy businessman for a large profit.

One week before the horse was to be sold, a hurricane swept through the farmer's land. It tore down the barn where the horse was kept and the stallion ran off.

"What bad luck!" the farmer's wife said.

"Good luck, bad luck, who knows, we'll have to see," said the farmer.

The next week, the farmer and his wife saw a herd of horses galloping toward the farm. There was their stallion, leading four horses behind him.

"What good luck!" said the farmer's wife.

"Good luck, bad luck, who knows, we'll have to see," said the farmer.

Soon the farmer and his son were training the new horses. One day the son was thrown by one of the horses and broke both his legs.

The farmer's wife was very upset. "My only son! We never should have let those horses in. This is very bad luck," she said.

"Good luck, bad luck, who knows, we'll have to see," said the farmer.

The next week soldiers came to the farm. Their king had declared war, and the soldiers were drafting every young man in the country. After seeing the farmer's son with both legs broken, the soldiers left him at home.

The farmer's wife was relieved, "Oh what good luck we have!"

As expected, the farmer said, "Good luck, bad luck, let's wait and see..."

This story illustrates how the farmer was a yogi in his understanding of change, staying detached from life's ups and downs. Change is the only thing we can be sure of, so why not accept it?

Let's accept and be thankful for what is true in our bodies and our minds at this moment, on this day. And know that change can be just a breath away.

Notes

Opening the Left Channel

Intention: To open the left nostril and activate the right brain.
Approximate Length: 3-5 minutes with breathing practice.

Do you ever come to class feeling agitated or unclear?

When we can begin our practice in a relaxed manner, it sanctions the right hemisphere of the brain, the part that handles music, color, complex memory, images and holistic thinking to function more fully and to integrate more readily with the left hemisphere — the side of the brain that handles rational thinking, external energies, and heat-inducing activities, such as digestion.

There are two channels which weave vital energy through the *chakras* in the spinal column, ending in either nostril, the *ida* (left) and *pingala* (right). When the breath is carried predominately through the left, *prana* flows through the channel that keeps the body calm and the mind quiet but alert. This is the ideal setting in which to practice *asana*.

Today we're going to begin our practice by opening the left nostril, the nostril that's responsible for activating the right brain.

Lie down on the right side, resting your right ear against the inner side of your upper arm. Stay here until the left nostril clears.

Each breath is like an ocean wave, swelling and receding again and again in perfect rhythm. Our yoga practice affords us the time to concentrate on this vital flow of nourishing air into and out of our bodies. Visualize a slow rolling ocean wave as you breathe completely and effortlessly.

Practice for Immune System

Intention: To integrate immune system enhancing practices into a traditional *asana* practice.
Approximate Length: 60 minutes with *asana/pranayama* practice.

Most of us get a cold or flu once or twice a year. However, if you're constantly getting sick, it could be a sign of an exhausted or lowered immune system.

The *chakra* most related to the immune system is *manipura chakra* at the solar plexus. This *chakra* relates to the adrenal glands. If the adrenals are overworked, our immune system will be weakened. The most important aspect for the health of *manipura* is to relieve stress and help the body to relax.

To boost your immune system include some *asanas* that work the *manipura chakra* along with *agni sara pranayama* and 2 to 1 breathing, drink 8 to 10 glasses of water a day and eat a diet rich in fiber to help the flow of food and toxins through the intestines. Include Vitamin C and zinc with your daily supplements, and get plenty of sleep.

Asana Practice for the Immune System

Surya Namaskara (sun salutation). 1-3 times

Agni Sara. 3-5 rounds (see p. 109)

Fire Series (leg lifts)

Dhanurasana (bow). Balances *agni* (internal fire), 2-3 times with **Child's Pose**.

Paschimottanasana (posterior stretch). Eliminates accumulated toxins, boosts immune system and improves circulation.

Twists. Helps the cleansing process, 1-3 times each side.

Sarvangasana (shoulderstand). Has a soothing effect on the nerves. Helps hypertension and insomnia.

2 to 1 Breathing. 2-3 minutes (see p. 52)

Shavasana/relaxation. 5-10 minutes

Asanas

Surya Namaskara
sun salutation
(see p.101 for basic 12 poses)

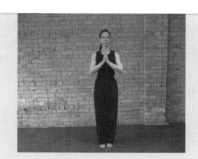

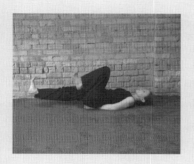

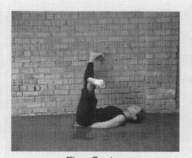

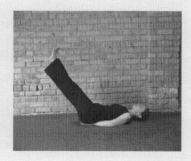

bicycling

Fire Series
spread leg stretch

double leg lifts

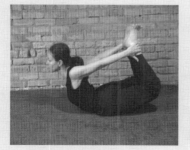

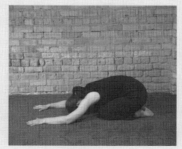

Dhanurasana
bow

Child's Pose

253

Asanas

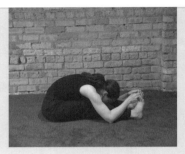

Paschimottanasana
posterior stretch

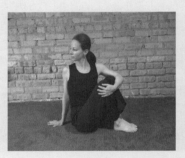
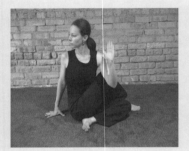

Seated Twists

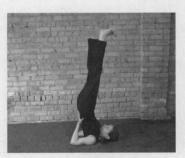

Sarvangasana
shoulderstand

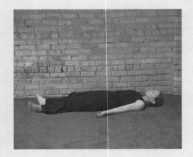

Shavasana
corpse

Silent Chanting

Intention: To silently purify the emotions.
Approximate Length: 5-6 minutes with chanting practice.

During the course of our busy days, it's tempting to fall mindlessly into noisy distractions that take us away from our true selves. Many of us find we need to fill the gaps of silence with the noise of radio, television and talk. We've become afraid of silence, like children afraid of the dark.

When we absorb our mind in chant, the sound that's produced by the body in union with the mind, we experience a purifying tool of the mind. Chant develops our concentration, strength of mind and purifies negative emotions. The intentional sound of chant rather than the noisy fillers of life enhance the silence around us, balance our inner and outer worlds, and take us back to our true selves.

The practice of chanting can integrate both silence and chant. This is referred to as "silent chanting." As a result, chanting can be practiced anywhere at anytime.

Applying a 3-part inhale, we can repeat the three seed syllables found in *om* (aum) silently in unison with our breathing: *Oh* is the seed sound of divine body, *Ah* is the seed sound of divine speech, and *M* is the seed sound of divine thought.

To practice silent chant, inhale the first third of your breath from pubic bone to navel and mentally say *Oh*. Inhale the second third of your breath from navel to heart and mentally say *Ah*. Finally, inhale the last third of your breath from heart to throat center and mentally say *M*, allowing the internal "mmmm" vibration to continue silently until the last bit of inhale is absorbed. Follow this inhale with an equally long and silent exhale of *om* from throat center to pubic bone.

Feel how the breath connects with the individual and divine body, speech and mind.

Think of these syllables as the universal embodiment of strength, openness and oneness.

Finally, allow your silent chanting to dissolve into relaxed breathing.

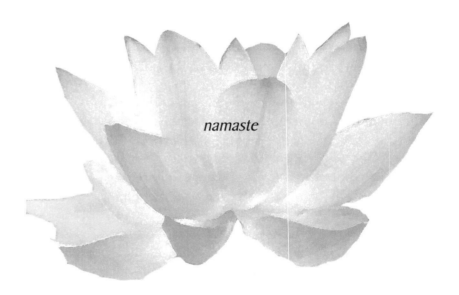

namaste

Recommended Reading

This list is merely a drop in the literary ocean of yoga knowledge and guidance.
These just happen to be some of my favorites.

Anderson, Sandra and Rolf Solvik, Psy.D. *Yoga: Mastering the Basics.* Honesdale, PA: The Himalayan Institute Press, 2000.

Arya, Usharbudh, Ph.D. *Philosophy of Hatha Yoga*, Glenview, IL: Himalayan International Institute of Yoga Science & Philosophy of USA, 1977.

Birch, Beryl Bender. *Beyond Power Yoga.* New York, NY: Fireside, 2000.

Brazier, David. *Zen Therapy: Transcending the Sorrows of the Human Mind.* New York, NY: John Wiley and Sons, Inc., 1995.

Easwaran, Eknath. (Translation) *The Upanishads.* Berkeley, CA: Blue Mountain Center of Meditation, 1987.

Farhi, Donna. *The Breathing Book.* New York, NY: Henry Holt and Company, 1996.

Feuerstein, Georg, Ph.D. *The Shambhala Encyclopedia of Yoga* Boston, MA: Shambhala Publications, Inc., 1997.

Feuerstein, Georg, Ph.D. (Translation and Commentary) *The Yoga Sutra of Patanjali.* Rochester, VT: Inner Traditions International, 1979, 1989.

Gates, Rolf and Katrina Kenison. *Meditations From the Mat.* New York, NY: Anchor Books, 2002.

Hanh, Thich Nhat.*Old Path White Clouds.* Berkeley, CA: Parallax Press, 1991.

Iyengar, B.K.S. *Light on Pranayama.* New York, NY: The Crossroad Publishing Co., 1998.

Iyengar, B.K.S. *Light on Yoga.* New York, NY: Schocken Books, 1979.

Iyengar, B.K.S. *Yoga: The Path to Holistic Health.* Great Britain: Dorling Kindersley Limited, 2001.

Johnsen, Linda. *Meditation Is Boring: Putting Life In Your Spiritual Practice.* Honesdale, PA: Himalayan Institute Press, 2000.

Kabat-Zinn, John, Ph.D. *Full Catastrophe Living.* New York, NY: Dell Publishing, 1991.

Kraftsow, Gary. *Yoga for Wellness.* New York, NY: The Penguin Group, 1999.

Lasater, Judith. *Living Your Yoga: Finding the Spiritual in Everyday Life.* Berkeley, CA: Rodmell Press, 2000.

Lowndes, Florin. *Enlivening the Chakra of the Heart.* Great Britain: Sophia Books, 1998.

Judith, Anodea. *Wheels of Life.* St. Paul, MN: Llewellyn Publications, 1998.

Mehta, Silva, Mira Mehta and Shyam Mehta. *Yoga: The Iyengar Way.* New York, NY: Alfred A. Knoff, 1997.

Myss, Caroline. *Anatomy of the Spirit.* New York, NY: Harmony Books, 1996.

Osho. *Meditation: The First and Last Freedom.* New York, NY: St. Martin's Griffin, 1997.

Prabhavananda, Swami and Christopher Isherwood, *Bhagavad Gita: The Song of God.* Hollywood, CA: Vedanta Press, 1978.

Prabhavananda, Swami and Christopher Isherwood, *How to Know God.* Hollywood, CA: Vedanta Press, 1981.

Rama., Swami *Living With the Himalayan Masters.* Honesdale, PA: Himalayan Institute Press, 1979, 1999.

Rama, Swami. *Meditation and Its Practice*. Honesdale, PA: Himalayan International Institute of Yoga Science and Philosophy, 1992.

Rama, Swami. *Path of Fire and Light*. Honesdale, PA: Himalayan International Institute of Yoga Science and Philosophy, 1986.

Rama, Swami, Rudolph Ballentine, M.D. and Alan Hymes,M.D. *Science of Breath*. Honesdale, PA: Himalayan Institute of Yoga Science and Philosophy, 1979.

Schaeffer, Rachel. *Yoga For Your Spiritual Muscles*. Wheaton, IL: Quest Books. 1998.

Schatz, Mary Pulling, M.D. *Back Care Basics*. Berkeley, CA: Rodmell Press, 1992.

Schiffman, Erich. *Yoga: The Spirit and Practice of Moving Into Stillness*. New York, NY: Pocket Books, 1996.

Shunryu,Suzuki. *Zen Mind, Beginner's Mind*. New York, NY: Beacon Press, 1996.

Thondup, Tulku. *The Healing Power of Mind*. Boston, MA: Shambhala Publications, 1996.

Tigunait, Pandit Rajmani, Ph.D. *At The Eleventh Hour*. Honesdale, PA: Himalayan Institute Press, 2001.

Tigunait, Pandit Rajmani., Ph.D. *The Power of Mantra and The Mystery of Initiation*. Honesdale, PA: Yoga International Books, 1996.

Vishnu-devananda, Swami. *The Complete Illustrated Book of Yoga*. New York, NY: Harmony Books. 1988.

Vishnu-devananda , Swami. Commentary. *Hatha Yoga Pradipika,* New York, NY: OM Lotus Publishing Company, 1987.

Yogananda, Paramahansa. *Autobiography of a Yogi*. Los Angeles, CA: Self-Realization Fellowship, 1998.

Glossary

Adho Mukha Shvanasana *(AH-doh MOO-kah shvah-NAH-sah-nah)* Downdog pose.

Agni Sara *(AHG-nee SAH- rah)* Yogic fire ignited by breathing practices.

Ajna *(AHJ-nah)* Sixth chakra located a the eyebrow center.

Ahimsa *(Ah-HIM- sah)* Non-harming.

Anahata *(Ohn-ah-HAH-tah)* Fourth chakra located at the heart center.

Anuloma Krama *(Ahn-ah-LOH-mah KRAH-mah)* Segmented inhalation.

Aparigraha *(Ah-PAH-ree-GRAH-hah)* Non-possessiveness.

Ardha Baddha Padma Paschimottanasana *(AHR-dah BAH-dah PAHD-mah Pash-ee-moh-tah-NAH-sah-nah)* Half-bound lotus posterior stretch.

Ardha Chandrasana *(AHR-dah Shahn-DRAH-sah-nah)* Half moon pose.

Asana *(AH-sah-nah)* Postures or yoga poses; third limb of Raja Yoga.

Asteya *(Ah-STAY-ah)* Non-stealing.

Asvini Mudra *(AHS-vee-nee MOO-drah)* Horse mudra.

Ashtanga *(AHSH-tahn-gah)* The eight limbs of Yoga as described by Patanjali.

Avidya *(Ah-VEED-yah)* Spiritual tunnel vision; ignorance.

Baddha Konasana (BAH-dah Koh-NAH-sah-nah) Bound angle or butterfly pose.

Chakra *(Shah-KRAH)* Spinning vortex of subtle energy.

Chakrasana *(Shah-KRAH-sah-nah)* Wheel pose.

Chaturanga *(Chaht-uh- RAHN-gah)* Stick or four limbs pose.

Dhanurasana *(Dohn-your-AH-sah-nah)* Bow pose.

Dharana *(Dah-RAH-nah)* Concentration; the sixth limb of Raja Yoga.

Dhyana *(Dee-YAH-nah)* Meditation; the seventh limb of Raja Yoga.

Drishti *(DRISH-tee)* Focus Point.

Garudasana *(Gah-roo-DAH-sah-nah)* Eagle pose.
Gomukhasana *(Goh-moo-KHA-sah-nah)* Cow's face pose.

Halasana *(Hah-LAH-sah-nah)* Plow pose.
Ham *(Hum)* Seed sound of the fifth chakra.
Hanumanasana *(Hah-new-mahn-AHS-ana)* Splits pose.
Hatha Yoga *(HAH-tah YOH-gah)* The physical practice of balancing the solar and lunar currents of human consciousness representing the dual nature of man.

Ida *(EE-dah)* The main energy channel that ends in the left nostril, embodying the moon, and connecting to right brain activity.
Ishvara Pranidhana *(ISH-var-ah PRAH-nee-DAH-nah)* Surrender to divine consciousness.

Janu Shirshana *(JAH-noo Shur-SHAH-sah-nah)* Head-to-knee pose.
Jathara Parivartanasana *(Jah-TAH-rah Pah-ree-var-TAHN-ah-sah-nah)* Leg lifts with twist.

Kapalabhati *(Kah-pah-lah-BHA-tee)* Shining skull breath using controlled but forceful exhalations.
Kapotasana *(Kah-POH-tah-sah-nah)* Pigeon pose.
Kundalini *(KOON-dah-lee-nee)* Dormant energy at the base of the spine awakened through various yoga practices.
Kurmasana *(Koohr-MAH-sah-nah)* Tortoise pose.

Lam *(Lum)* Seed sound of the first chakra.

Makarasana *(MAHK-ah-RAH-sah-nah)* Crocodile pose.
Manipura *(Mahn-ah-PUR-ah)* Third chakra located at the solar plexus.
Mantra *(MAHN-trah)* Sacred sound used in meditation.
Marichyasana *(MAH-rih-si-AH-sah-nah)* Seated Twist.
Matsyasana *(Mahtz-YAH-sah-nah)* Fish pose.
Muladhara *(MOO-lah-hah-rah)* Root chakra located at the perineum.
Mula Bandha *(MOO-lah BAHN-dah)* Root lock.

Nadi *(NAH-dee)* Subtle energy channel.

Nadi Shodhana *(NAH-dee Shoh-DAH-nah)* Alternate nostril breathing.

Namaste *(Nah-MAHS-tay)* The light in me bows to the light in you.

Natarajasana *(Nah-tah-raj-AH-sah-nah)* King dancer pose.

Naukasana *(Now-KAH-sah-nah)* Reclining boat pose.

Navasana *(Nah-VAH-sah-nah)* Sitting boat balance pose.

Niyamas *(Nee-YAH-mahs)* Observances; the second limb of Raja Yoga.

Om *(Ohm)* Divine sound of the universe.

Padmasana *(PAHD-mah-sah-nah)* Lotus pose.

Patanjali *(Pah-TAHN-joh-lee)* Hindu Sage and author of the *Yoga Sutras*.

Parivrtta Janu Sirasana *(Par-ee-vrit-ah JAH-noo Shur-SHAH-sah-nah)* Revolved head to knee pose.

Parivrtta Trikonasana *(Par-ee-vrit-ah Trik-cohn-AH-sah-nah)* Revolved triangle pose.

Paschimottanasana *(POSH-ee-moh-tah-NAH-sah-nah)* Posterior stretch pose.

Parshvakonasana *(Par-shvah-KOH-nah-sah-nah)* Triangle II pose or Side Angle pose.

Parshvottanasana *(Par-shvot-TAH-nah-sah-nah)* Angle or Pyramid pose.

Pingala *(Peen-GAH-lah)* The main energy channel that ends in the right nostril, embodies the sun, and is connected to left brain activity.

Prana *(PRAH-nah)* Universal energy that animates all living things.

Pranayama *(PRAH-nah-YAH-mah)* Control of lifeforce; also referred to as breathing exercises; fourth limb of Raja Yoga.

Prasarita Padottanasana *(Prah-sa-REE-tah Pah-doh-tahn-AH-sah-nah)* Standing spread leg forward bend.

Pratyahara *(PRAH-tyah-HAH-rah)* Withdrawal of the senses; fifth limb of Raja Yoga.

Raja Yoga *(RHA-jah YO-gah)* The Royal Path; eight-limbed path of yoga.

Ram *(Rum)* Seed sound of the third chakra.

Sahasrara *(Sah-haz-RAH-rah)* Seventh chakra located at the crown of the head.

Samadhi *(Sah-MAH-dee)* The super-conscious state, a state of bliss; the eighth limb of *Raja* Yoga.

Santosha *(San-TOH-shah)* Contentment.

Sarvangasana *(SAHR-vahn-GAH-sah-nah)* Shoulderstand.

Saucha *(Soh-shah)* Purity.

Satya *(SAHT-yah)* Truth.

Setu Bandha Sarvangasana *(SAY-too BAHN-dah SAHR-vahn-GAH-sah-nah)* Bridge pose.

Shalabhasana *(Shah-lah-BAH-sah-nah)* Locust pose.

Shanti *(SHAHN-tee)* Peace.

Shavasana *(Shah-VAH-sah-nah)* Corpse pose.

Simhasana *(Sim-HAH-sah-nah)* Lion pose.

Shirshasana *(Sher-SHAH-sah-nah)* Headstand.

Sukhasana *(Soo- KAH-sah- nah)* Easy pose.

Supta Sukhasana *(Soop-TAH Soo-KAH-sah-nah)* Reclining easy pose.

Surya Namaskara *(SOOR-yah Nah-mahs-KAH-rah)* Sun Salutation.

Sushumna *(Soo-SHOOM-nah)* The central and main nadi that runs along the spine and ends at the crown chakra.

Svadhisthana *(SVAHD- hiss-tahn-ah)* Second chakra located at the lower abdomen.

Svadhyaya *(Svahd-YAH-yah)* Self-study.

Tadasana *(Ta-DAH-sah-nah)* Mountain pose.

Tapas *(TAH-pahs)* Determined effort.

Tittibhasana *(Tee-tah-BAH-SAH-nah)* Firefly pose.

Trikonasana *(Trik-cohn-AH-sah-nah)* Triangle pose.

Uddiyana Bandha *(OO-DEE-anna BAHN-dah)* An energy lock that includes a forceful exhalation followed by a sharp sucking up of the intestines and diaphragm into a vacuum created in the thoracic cavity.

Ujjayi *(OO-JAH-yee)* A breathing practice that uses an audible vibration by gently closing the glottis in the throat.

Upavistha Konasana *(Oo-pah-VEESH-tah Kohn-NAH-sah-nah)* Seated angle pose.

Urdhva Mukha Shvanasana *(OORD-vah MOOK-hah Shvah-NAH-sah- nah)* Upward facing dog pose.

Ustrasana *(Oohs-TRAH-sah-nah)* Camel pose.

Uttanasana *(OOH-tah-NAH-sah-nah)* Standing forward bend.

Vam *(Vum)* Seed sound of the second chakra.

Vasishthasana *(Vah-shish-TAHS-ah-nah)* Side plank pose

Vinyasa *(Vin-YAH-sah)* A series of asanas linking movement with breath.

Virabhadrasana *(Veer-ah-bah-DRAH-sah-nah)* Warrior pose.

Virasana *(Vir-AH-sah-nah)* Hero pose.

Visuddha *(Vah-SHOE-dah)* Fifth chakra located at the throat center.

Vrikshasana *(Vrik-SHAH-sah-nah)* Tree pose.

Vrittis *(Vrit-EEZ)* Fluctuations of the mind.

Yamas (YAH-mahs) Five restraints; first limb of Raja Yoga.

Yoga *(YOH-gah)* To join or yoke.

Yoga Sutras *(YOH-gah SOOT-rahs)* A series of aphorisms relating to the practice of yoga as codified by Patanjali.

Index

C

U

about the author

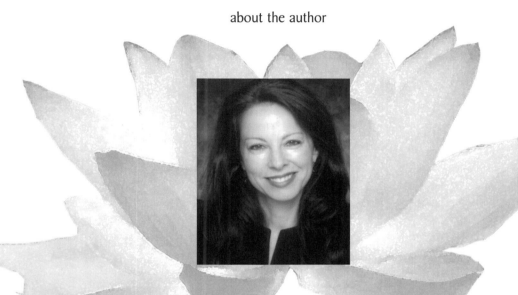

Nancy Gerstein is a Certified Hatha Yoga Teacher with the Himalayan Institute of Yoga Philosophy and Science, a Reiki Master-Practitioner, yoga therapist and frequent workshop speaker.

Ms. Gerstein's teaching emphasis takes the ancient lessons of yoga philosophy and integrates them into daily living. She believes that to live a more joyous life, yoga practice cannot end when we leave the classroom and can often be heard telling her students to go out and live their yoga.

For further information on Ms. Gerstein's classes and workshops, please contact her at authors@pendragonpublishinginc.com or guidingyogaslight.com.